'EDUCATION E LIBRARY'
ROYAL INFIRMARY

KV-195-395

This book is to be returned on or before
the last date stamped below.

HISTORY OF MEDICINE

DR BEHR ROOM
MACKENZIE HEALTHCARE LIBRARY
BURNLEY GENERAL HOSPITAL

HISTORY 25/2/2

CLASS No.   610.9

AUTHOR: SYKES, W.S.

BURNLEY MACKENZIE
HEALTHCARE LIBRARY

TU05848

TITLE: Essays on the first
       hundred years of
       anaesthesia   (555)

"EDUCATION OF THE LIBRARY"
ROYAL INFIRMARY BLACKBURN

ESSAYS ON THE
FIRST HUNDRED YEARS
OF ANÆSTHESIA

TO NAN

who pushed me into this labour of Hercules in the first place; and who helped, loved, cherished and over-fed me through the joyous and delightful years of its fulfilment;

AND IN MEMORY OF
MY FATHER

who had a cholecystectomy done by a most skilful surgeon, with all the ritual, panoply, safety and security of modern surgery, . . . and died thereafter.

AND IN MEMORY OF
HER FATHER,

to whom exactly the same tragic thing happened.

In the hope that this work may help indirectly towards safer surgery. For the value of history lies in the fact that we learn by it from the mistakes of others. Learning from our own is a slow process.

"EDUCATION OF THE LIBRARY"
ROYAL INFIRMARY BLACKBURN

TB02010

ESSAYS ON THE FIRST HUNDRED YEARS OF ANÆSTHESIA

by

W. STANLEY SYKES,

M.B.E., M.B., B.Chir. (Cantab.), D.A.

Late Anæsthetist to the General Infirmary at Leeds, to the Hospital for Women and St. James' Hospital, Leeds, to the Leeds Dental Hospital, to the Halifax Royal Infirmary and to the Dewsbury General Hospital.

Volume 1

CHURCHILL LIVINGSTONE
EDINBURGH LONDON MELBOURNE AND NEW YORK 1982

CHURCHILL LIVINGSTONE
Medical Division of Longman Group Limited

Distributed in the United States of America and Canada
by the American Society of Anesthesiologists Inc.,
515 Busse Highway, Park Ridge, Illinois 60068.
Distributed elsewhere throughout the world by Churchill
Livingstone and associated companies, branches and
representatives.

© E. & S. Livingstone Limited 1960
© Longman Group Limited 1982

All rights reserved. No part of this publication
may be reproduced, stored in a retrieval system,
or transmitted in any form or by any means,
electronic, mechanical, photocopying, recording
or otherwise, without the prior permission of the
publishers (Churchill Livingstone, Robert Stevenson
House, 1–3 Baxter's Place, Leith Walk,
Edinburgh, EH1 3AF).

First published 1960
Reprinted 1982

ISBN 0 443 02823 0

British Library Cataloguing in Publication Data
Sykes, W. Stanley
    Essays on the first hundred years of anaesthesia.
    Vol. 1
    1. Anesthesia—History
    I. Title
    617'.96'09   RD79

EDUCATION CENTRE
LIBRARY
ACC. No. 820622
CLASS No. 610.9

Printed in Great Britain by
William Clowes (Beccles) Limited,
Beccles and London

BURIALS in the Parish of _Winlaton_
in the County of _Durham_ ___ in the Year 184_

Name.	Abode.	When buried.	Age.	By whom the Ceremony was performed.
Isabella Atkinson No. 1089.	Winlaton	Jany. 12.	85 years	Charles Tinley
John Golightly No. 1090.	Shew	Jany 13	16 years	Charles Tinley
Hannah Greener No. 1091.	Winlaton	Jany 30.	15 years	Charles Tinley

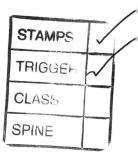

PLATE I

Entry in the Register of Burials for the Parish of Winlaton, County Durham. Photographed by the author in the Rectory of the Parish Church, by permission of the Rector of Winlaton, 1958.

This was the first recorded death under anæsthesia, on 28th January, 1848. Hannah Greener, of Winlaton, aged 15, died under chloroform and was buried on 30th January, after an inquest.

Note the marginal entry, "Died from effects of chloriform". The Rev. Charles Tinley can be pardoned for his spelling mistake. The word was not then as familiar to the lay public as it was later. Dr. Meggison, of Whickham, a village about half a mile away, was the anæsthetist. Mr. Lloyd, his assistant, was going to remove an ingrowing toe nail. Death was quite sudden, under very light chloroform anæsthesia in the sitting position.

Unfortunately there is no plan or record of Hannah's grave in the churchyard. Nan and I searched for a long time without success. At the cost of many nettle stings and thistle scratches we found the graves of other Greeners, but not Hannah's.

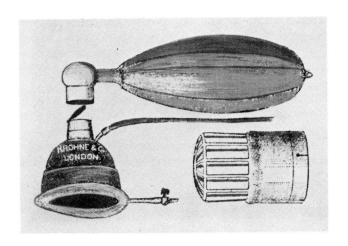

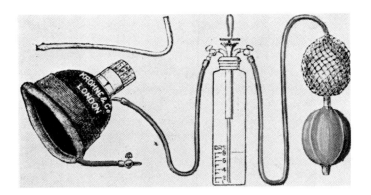

PLATE II

"Some are gentle, like the little hinged feather used as a breathing indicator."
Lancet, 1894, Nov. 3. 1038. Krohne and Sesemann's regulating inhalers for chloroform and ether. The chloroform inhaler is an ordinary Junker's inhaler with a facepiece fitted with a feather in a protective cage as a breathing indicator, double taps and a filling funnel. The ether inhaler uses the same facepiece with the cage removed and a bag added, also a larger bottle (2 oz.) with a bone terminal to the tube which dips into the ether, to prevent freezing. *The Lancet* does not think that this will be as satisfactory as the chloroform inhaler, but recommends it for A.C.E. mixture. They also criticise the taps, which were added so that the remaining chloroform could be kept for the next case. *The Lancet* says that it should be thrown away, and also points out that the inhaler can be put together wrongly.

PREFACE

"It is for us, the living, rather to be dedicated here to the unfinished work
which they who fought here have thus so nobly advanced. It is rather for us
to be here dedicated to the great task remaining before us, that . . . we here
highly resolve that these dead shall not have died in vain".

—ABRAHAM LINCOLN, *Gettysburg speech,* 1863.

SOME of the apparatuses and devices illustrated here are severely
practical; some are so theoretical as to remind you of the White
Knight in Alice in Wonderland. His sandwich box, you will
remember, was slung upside down, so that the rain couldn't get in. This
had the disadvantage that the sandwiches always fell out, but the box
did keep dry inside.

Some are simplicity itself, others most damnably complicated. Some
are ingenious, others plain stupid; some are very essential, others highly
unnecessary. Some are as safe as it is possible for a machine to be, others
quite frankly dangerous. Some are clever, others can only be described
as the lunatic fringe. Some are gentle, like the little hinged feather used
as a breathing indicator on some early Junker's inhaler masks. Others
are brutal, like Heister's mouth opener, which is really only suitable for
removing refractory wheels from old railway trucks.

I began this book on an extensive scale, with the object of photographing them all—everything connected in any way with anæsthesia,
or employed by anæsthetists, or which might suggest anything useful to
anæsthetists. My object was to make a comprehensive encyclopædia, in
which anybody who comes across an antique machine could identify it
with certainty; in which anyone who is designing an apparatus could
find out how often his new and original ideas have been used before; and
in which anyone could browse and find something new. It was planned
on a scale suggestive of the *Encyclopædia Britannica* or Gibbon's *Decline and
Fall of the Roman Empire.*

Like the compiler of a dictionary, I did not intend to omit things
because I don't like them, or because I don't use them, or because I don't
agree with them. It would be a stupid and useless dictionary which did
this. After all, people still want to look the words up, even if the compiler
doesn't like them.

Moreover, the collection would not be limited to anæsthetic apparatus, strictly so-called; it would include resuscitation methods of all kinds—oxygen apparatus, blood transfusion and all accessories such as gags, airways, intratracheal tubes and tracheotomy tubes; in fact, anything

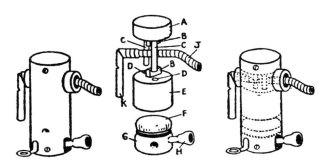

FIG. 1

One of "the two devices which blow a whistle when the gas cylinder is running out in the darkness of the X-ray room."

Lancet, 1943, Oct. 16. 481. W. H. Marshall. Audible warning of empty gas cylinders. The apparatus is made out of scrap material. The "saucepan" G is surmounted by a thin rubber diaphragm F, which rises when fed with gas from a reducing valve at 5 lb. pressure. The diaphragm balloons upwards and raises the plunger E. This nips the tube J, which feeds the whistle, between the blunt knife edges B and B. The whistle K, which is supplied with air from a Junker's bulb, is then unable to sound. When the gas pressure falls the plunger E also falls and the whistle sounds. The rods C work in the holes D to compel the rising knife edge on the plunger B to keep vertically in line with its mate on the fixed member A.

which can be or has been of use to or of interest to the anæsthetist. After all, resuscitation has always been very much a part of the anæsthetist's job, from that tragic day in 1848 when Hannah Greener died under the hands of Dr. Meggison to the present day. It always will be part of his job.

So I began to go relentlessly through the literature, photographing every apparatus I came across. It proved to be an enormous task. I have collected nearly 6,000 of them. There will be some duplication, no doubt, in such a colossal collection, but even after extensive pruning there

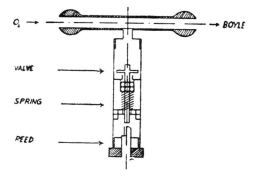

Fig. 2

Another device to give warning of empty cylinders. Useful in darkened theatres.

Brit. med. J., 1943, Oct. 30. 548. Massey Dawkins. As soon as the gas flow is less than 5 lb. per sq. in. pressure, the spring pushes up the valve and allows gas to escape through the reed. The spring is adjustable. Can be used for any gas. Made by Medical and Industrial Equipment Co., Ltd.

Again, both these contrivances have been anticipated. *Lancet, 1868, Dec. 12. 780.* Mr. Porter (of J. Bell & Co.) described a generator for nitrous oxide which had two novel features. This was just before gas cylinders came into use, when you had to make your own gas. It had a temperature regulator by which, as the temperature and with it the pressure increased, water was forced up a tube, raising a float which acted on a lever to shut down the coal gas supply to the burner under the retort.

Also, if the storage bag or gasometer was full, a whistle blew, as a warning to stop the process before something blew up. No illustration was given.

Lancet, 1907, June 29. 1769. Lieut. Vaugînot designed a breathing apparatus for the Sapeurs-Pompiers (Fire Brigade), in which a whistle blew when the oxygen pressure fell below a certain level. This was not illustrated.

A safety device of this sort would probably have prevented part of a recent tragedy. The reference is to an ex-consultant anæsthetist who acquired the habit of inhaling the anæsthetic himself. During the semi-stupor produced by this an oxygen cylinder ran out and the patient, a child, died on the table.

The anæsthetist lost his job, got a gaol sentence and was struck off the register. The persistent whistle of an expiring cylinder fitted with one of these gadgets would at least have roused the theatre staff to do something about it at an earlier stage, while there was yet time. It would have saved the patient, if not the anæsthetist.

will remain well over five thousand. At the same time I looked at every reference to anæsthesia in the whole hundred years of *The Lancet* and many in other journals, and abstracted most of them into a card index.

Some of the early illustrations were very bad and blotchy, especially the early half-tone blocks, which were much worse than their predecessors the woodcuts. The copies of these suffered accordingly. In many old weekly journals, which have rested on library shelves for over a hundred years, the ink on the reverse side of the pages showed through the paper, which itself was very far from white by this time. This again did not help in getting good copies. Given good originals I could get clear reproductions.

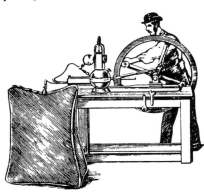

FIG. 3

"For charm I give the first place to the little man in the bowler hat. . . ."

Breathing in Irrespirable Atmospheres. Sir Robert H. Davis. (Not dated, but from internal evidence, probably about 1947). The manufacture and storage of oxygen in the very early 20th century. It was made by heating a mixture of potassium chlorate and the catalyst manganese dioxide, or by Brin's process, in which barium oxide (BaO) is heated in air to red heat with the formation of barium peroxide (BaO2). This took place at 500°C The heating was continued to 800°C (white heat), when the compound decomposed into the oxide and oxygen. The steel cylinder was not available at this time, so the containers were made of copper, and the maximum pressure allowed was 30 atmospheres or 450 lb. per sq. in. The oxygen was first collected in a bag which was attached to the suction side of pump by which it was compressed into the cylinder by the exertions of the man in the bowler hat.

The three previous best books as regards illustrations of old anæsthetic apparatus are Barbara Duncum's *Development of Inhalation Anæthesia* (1947), Oxford University Press, which shows about 142 of them, and *The Principles of Thoracic Anæsthesia,* by W. W. Mushin and L. Rendell-Baker (1953), Blackwell, Oxford, which shows just over 200. Noel Gillespie's *Endotracheal Anæsthesia* (1941, 1948), University of Wisconsin Press, has 56 illustrations. Other histories are very sparsely illustrated. Thomas Keys, with his 1,200 references, gives exactly five pictures of apparatus. Bankoff illustrates one only, as does Fülöp-Miller.

My ideal is a book which includes pictures of every apparatus which has ever been used in anæsthesia, a book whose compilation involves going through everything which has ever been written about anæsthesia during its first hundred years. It is an impossible task, but one can at least aim at it. It has, so far, meant going

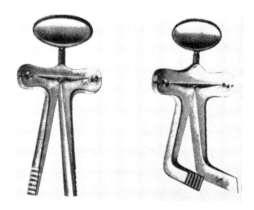

PLATE III

"Others are brutal, like Heister's mouth opener, which is really only suitable for removing refractory wheels from old railway trucks".

Handbuch der allgemeinen und lokalen Anæsthesie. Prof. Dr. F. L. Dumont, Bern., 1903.

Heister's gag, straight and bent models. A fearsome object of tremendous leverage. In the catalogue of Salt & Son of Birmingham it is called Clover's gag, but I think Clover was far too good an anæsthetist to design such a destructive and terrible instrument. In the catalogue of Archibald Young of Edinburgh it is called Newington's gag.

But there is no doubt that it is of Continental origin. At any rate I have never seen it in England (or America), whereas in the operating theatres in which I worked while a prisoner of war in Germany it appeared to be a standard fitting together with Roser-Koenig's gag.

Some evidence as to Clover's gentleness is given in: *Lancet, 1879, Nov. 1. 659.* Leading article on artificial respiration. "We have seen surgeons pull forward the tongue with forceps in cases of danger during the inhalation of anæsthetics, but we have always considered it a very rough proceeding, and we are glad to hear from Mr. Clover that the elevation of the chin is quite sufficient and altogether preferable".

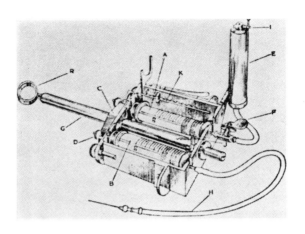

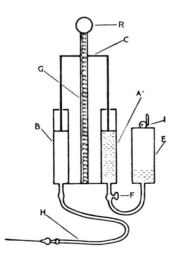

PLATE IV

"For sheer ingenuity the designs which appeal to me are . . ."

Brit. med. J., 1939, Mar. 4. 449. J. B. Devine, Melbourne. A slow motion, automatic syringe for giving small amounts over a period of time. Made by Ulrich of Ulm. Two standard 10 cc. syringes A and B have their plungers linked together by the bar C. Syringe B gives the injection, its rate of flow being controlled by syringe A. The flow of the latter is in its turn controlled by the screw tap F, the resistance of which regulates the release of the spring G, which exercises a constant pressure on the coupled pistons. I is an air vent. J is a clip which fixes the spring, while the tap F is regulated. The lever K catches on a serrated bar and clicks as each half cc. is injected. The nut D unscrews to allow of sterilisation. The injection of 10 cc. may be spread over an hour. If less is required the syringe B may be of smaller diameter than the control syringe and correspondingly less fluid will be given.

PLATE V

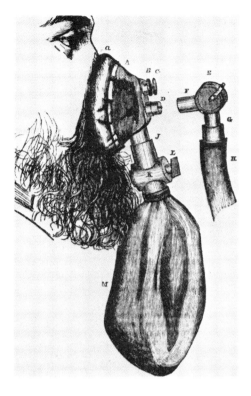

"My sympathies are entirely with Clover in his valiant efforts to give gas to heavily bearded gentlemen who must have leaked air in from every point of the compass."

Although beards could be useful on occasion. *Lancet, 1876, Oct. 14. 534.* Mr. Morton describes the case of a man of 44 who was to have an eye removed. Ether was given on a sponge, and his tongue and jaw fell back "but by forcibly pulling forward the lower jaw by means of his beard the patient was fully anæsthetised in about seven minutes after inhaling about five ounces of ether."

Brit. med. J., 1868, Nov. 7. 491. J. T. Clover. On the administration of nitrous oxide. This was the beginning of the renaissance of nitrous oxide in England, after T. W. Evans, the American dentist of Paris, had demonstrated it in London. He used a crude wooden mouthpiece and an assistant closed the nostrils. There was much struggling and some patients appeared to feel pain. Clover straightway improved the apparatus by a sheet lead facepiece edged with rubber tubing. M was a bag of 200 cubic inches. Clover remarked that sometimes the anæsthesia could be prolonged by his nosepiece from the chloroform apparatus. He reported 384 cases, mostly dentals, but including a few other minor operations. M is the supplemental bag. C expiratory valve. D mount on which the stopcock FG fits. The spindle part of the inspiratory valve is seen projecting. E air opening. When the little knob is turned down to G the air opening E is closed and the supply tube H is opened. L tap to shut off supplementary bag.

Joseph Thomas Clover was born Feb. 28, 1825. He qualified in 1844. He was certainly present at Liston's first operation under ether (*Lancet, 1882, Oct. 14. 649. Mr. Squire*). He became house surgeon to Mr. Morton and then to Syme, who offered him a post in Edinburgh when he returned there. Clover preferred to stay in London and was R.M.O. at University College Hospital in 1848. He then devoted himself entirely to anæsthetics and became chloroformist to Westminster and University College Hospitals and to the Dental Hospital.

He gave an anæsthetic to the Prince of Wales (later Edward VII) in 1877, for an abscess of the perineum, attributed to a hunting injury. He also gave chloroform to Napoleon III, at Chislehurst, on 2nd Jan., 1873. Sir Henry Thompson sounded, detected a stone in the bladder and crushed it. On 6th Jan. Clover anæsthetised him again for a second evacuation sitting. The ex-Emperor died on 9th Jan. Clover signed the post-mortem report on 10th Jan. with five others.

Clover died on Sept. 27, 1882, aged 57, leaving a widow and four children.

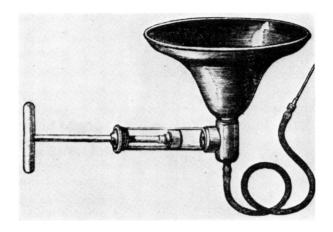

PLATE VI

Med. Times and Gazette, 1875, Oct. 30. 508.
Collin's transfusion apparatus. Made by
Salt & Son. Capacity of funnel 10 oz. A
float on the surface of the blood cuts off air
entry when the fluid is exhausted. A hard
rubber ball in the distribution chamber will
not allow blood to return to the funnel. But
if the chamber is empty this ball falls to the
end of the transfusion tube and closes it.
There are no sharp edged valves to cause
clotting. Air cannot be injected.

facing page 9

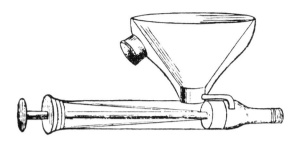

FIG. 4

"A fact which surprised me was the number of transfusion apparatuses designed by intrepid individuals who knew nothing . . . about blood grouping or even asepsis . . ."

Brit. med. J., 1858, Apr. 10. 290. John Wheatcroft. Transfusion apparatus. The donor is bled into the funnel and the blood is pumped into the recipient by the syringe. The funnel has a hot-water jacket. 18 ounces were successfully given to a woman moribund with post-partum haemorrhage. In another case 22 oz. were given successfully.

"The instrument in the drawing presents the following peculiarities: (*a*) The blood, being surrounded by hot water, is kept at a proper and even temperature; (*b*) The cup being firmly fixed to the syringe, the operator can hold it himself, and more readily proportion the supply of blood; (*c*) The thin film or sheet of India rubber, attached to the bottom of the piston-rod at one end and to the edge of the cylinder at the other, effectually prevents the injection of air, however careless the operator may be; (*d*) The mouth of the nozzle must be open, not crossed by a silver bar, as it usually is. For convenience of carriage, the cup should be made of vulcanised India-rubber.

This is somewhat similar to Collin's apparatus.

It was nine years before Lister began his campaign for cleanliness. Blood groups A, B and O were not known until 1900, when Landsteiner described them. In 1902 his pupils, Decastello and Sturli, found the rarest group AB. In 1911 the sub-groups of A were published by von Dungern and Hirszfield. Landsteiner and Levine identified the M, N and P groups in 1926. Landsteiner and Wiener identified the Rh system in 1940.

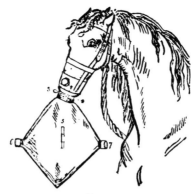

FIG. 5

The Pharmaceutical Journal for 1847 is full of pictures of
new ether apparatuses. I have no less than 29 of them from
that one volume alone. Mr. Hooper, who was very early
in the field with inhalers for human beings, also produced
a veterinary model.

Pharm. J., 1847, VII, Sept. 133. Mr. W. Hooper. Horse
inhaler for ether. 1, Muzzle; 2, Expiring valve; 3 and 4
Bayonet joint and inhaling valve; 5, Vulcanized India-
rubber bag; 6 and 7, Inhaling tubes. Directions: The
muzzle and vulcanized India-rubber (connected by a
bayonet joint) should be detached before being applied.
The *muzzle* is fixed to the horse by means of a head-piece
similar to a bridle, and a tight India-rubber band placed
over it near the top. The moveable brass piece underneath
the muzzle should be *closed*, and the *expiring* valve kept
open by the bent wire being placed underneath whilst
fixing it. The sponge in the vulcanized bag should be
taken out and soaked for a few seconds in *hot* water, and
then quickly wrung and put back into the bag, into which
is poured the ether. The bag should then be attached to
the muzzle. A strap in the front of the head-piece should
be passed through the loop in the bag, to prevent its col-
lapsing. The moveable brass piece to be *opened*, and the
bent wire underneath the *expiring valve* removed that the
valve may be set free. *In general the horse falls in about
three or five minutes, when the head should be quickly secured,
and according to the degree of stupor,* so must the expiring
valve be kept open, and the moveable brass piece closed
at the judgment of the operator.

Mr. Hooper was also early in the field as regards
oxygen administration. There was no picture of this,
but in *Pharm. J., 1847, VI, Apr., 508,* he described an
oxygen attachment which he had fitted to the Robinson
inhaler, for resuscitating etherised patients.

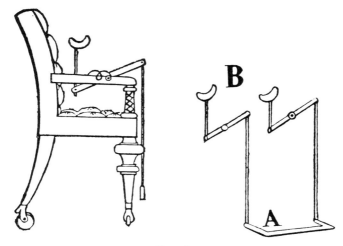

Fig. 6

Brit. med. J., 1869, Mar. 13. 235. Percy Leslie. Birmingham.
Artificial respiration apparatus. A chair fitted with a treadle,
which lifts the patient's arms. The dyspnoeic or collapsed
patient, who is already short of breath, or he would not be
needing artificial respiration, is apparently expected to pedal
like hell and do his own "assisted" breathing. Really, Mr.
Leslie! This is one of fifty methods of artificial respiration of
which I have photographs, but none of the others are as daft
as this.

through, page by page, over 1 million pages of medical journals and
over 50,000 pages in 211 text books and pamphlets. It was not sufficient
to rely on the indexes. This would have meant far too many omissions.

Pictures were copied with a Retina camera and copying stand. My
thanks are due to Mr. R. I. Cooper for developing and printing many
thousands of photographs, and for instructing me in a routine which
enabled me to get good copies easily and quickly. I have to thank the
Brotherton Library of the University of Leeds, and especially its branch
library at the Leeds Medical School for the loan of very many volumes.
As these libraries are only seven miles away they were very convenient of
access, and I am much indebted to the Librarian for allowing a non-
Leeds graduate to use them. In the first year I took 424 volumes out
from the Medical School Library. This was before I retired and was
part-time work only. The total is now over 900. The Library Inter-loan
scheme was also invaluable in obtaining some scarce items.

I have also to thank the University Library at Cambridge for the loan of many rare books. Some forty years after going down, when the idea of this book occurred to me (or to Nan, for she pushed me into it in the first place) I approached the mighty new building of this awe-inspiring Library with a certain amount of trepidation. On rather timidly enquiring whether I could use the Library, the assistant merely asked for my name and College and date of degree. He checked these in a printed volume and said at once, "Of course you can use it. It is *your* Library." A very charming and encouraging reception.

FIG. 7

Medical Record, 1900, Oct. 20. 601. J. Leonard Corning. New York. Spinal anæsthesia needle. (His first paper—the first ever on this subject —was in the *New York Medical Journal, 1885, Oct. 31.*) The needle is 3½-4 inches long, with a short bevel. It is made of gold or platina, which will not break. There is a small sliding nut with a setscrew to act as a distance piece. Also there is an introducer, many of which were introduced again many years later. Corning stresses asepsis. He used cocaine, 2% in doses of 10-15 minims. He kept the needle in position until the anæsthesia began, thus there was no leakage of cerebro-spinal fluid. Corning was a neurologist, not a surgeon. This was an extremely well-designed spinal needle. Many later ones were thick and clumsy, and lacked all the carefully thought-out features of this, the first, one.

Unfortunately Cambridge is 150 miles away and could only be visited rarely while I was still in general practice. So the near-by Leeds served as my mainstay. Postal libraries like Lewis's and the B.M.A. Library were also very useful.

Perhaps I should mention that I have been an anæsthetist myself for twenty-five years. I am a survivor from the stone age or bow and arrow epoch, by which I mean that I have never given a relaxant in my life. I gave up anæsthesia altogether at the end of World War II. During the last four years of my anæsthetic career—that is during the part of it which came into the relaxant era—I worked in German prisoner of war camps, where conditions were sometimes quite good, but refinements of this sort were absent. And so it came about that I was quite out of date when we returned home after being liberated by Patton's Third Army. So it seemed a good time to retire.

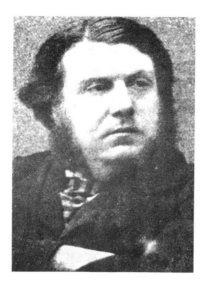

PLATE VII

".A merciless, truculent and pugnacious controversialist."

Brit. med. J., 1899, June 24. 1561. Lawson Tait, Birmingham gynæcologist and pioneer in ovariotomy. Born May 1, 1845. Qualified 1866. House surgeon in Wakefield, 1867. Did his first ovariotomy, July 29, 1868, at the age of 23. Surgeon to the Hospital for Women, Birmingham, 1871. Journalist, city councillor, good speaker and a controversial fighter. In 1884 completed his first 1,000 abdominal sections. In 1885 published 139 consecutive ovariotomies without a death. He tried Listerism and gave it up in favour of "asepsis"—a somewhat sketchy form of cleanliness. In 1894 he completed 4,000 abdominal sections.

Lancet, 1871, Jan. 14. 45. He describes some cases treated by Lister's method with bad results. "The difficulty cannot be got over by saying that the antiseptic precautions were not perfect. They were. I did all the dressings myself, and can assert that the Lister method . . . was carried out most faithfully. . . ." "My opinion of the antiseptic treatment is that its merits have been greatly exaggerated. . . ."

In 1895 (*Lancet, Sept. 21. 755*) he had a violent controversy with Sir Wm. Priestley about over-operating in gynæcology. The latter said that operating fees might influence the operator. Tait retaliates by mentioning a wealthy case attended by both of them, in which his advice of operation was refused. He said that, in this case, owing to prolonged attendance, he got about five times as much as he would have charged for an operation. Sir William, in a later letter, said that his facts about this case were all wrong. This has nothing to do with anæsthesia, so we must not follow this trail any longer.

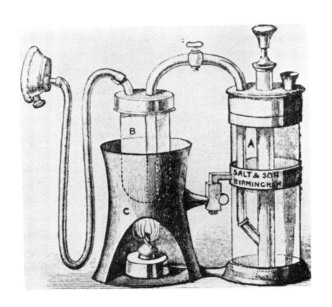

PLATE VIII

"As a designer of anæsthetic apparatus he cannot be given many marks."

Lancet, 1876, May 13. 721. Lawson Tait. Warm ether inhaler. Made by Salt & Son, Birmingham. Pure ether can be given at body temperature unmixed with air. Induction is more rapid and agreeable. "No risk of bronchitis, which is sometimes induced by the intense cold resulting from the vapourisation of ether." The inhaler was made of glass and metal. Ether was pumped from A to B, which is in a waterbath with a spirit lamp underneath. It is not stated how long this machine was in use before it blew up.

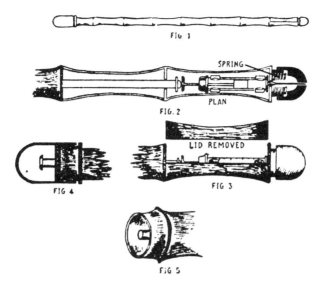

FIG. 8

Brit. med. J., 1941, Oct. 11. 513. A. Buchanan Barbour. A syringe made necessary by the advance of modern civilisation. Designed for injecting morphia into inaccessible victims trapped or buried during air raids. A six foot bamboo pole, with a syringe fixed at one end. A rod runs through the pole to a button at the other end. Push the button and the injection is made, through the clothes, six feet away.

In a book like this a reference could be attached to almost every sentence until the book itself became unreadable, its very sense and meaning lost and obscured by an inky snowdrift of footnotes. So references are only given when they are of some importance, and then they are segregated at the ends of the chapters. If I make some startling, some critical or some disparaging remark, there is usually a reference to support it. And there are criticisms in plenty, for there are many instances of crass stupidity, of distortion or suppression of facts in order to bolster up pre-conceived opinions, of rash statements without foundation, of foolish suggestions and dangerous ideas, of premature optimism and of fatuous self-complacency.

All these things have cost lives, and the value of history is that it may enable us to avoid making too often the mistakes that others have already made. But in order to avoid them it is essential to know about them. That is why history is of practical value to the anæsthetist.

I have tried to concentrate upon subjects which have been dealt with inadequately or not dealt with at all by other historians. I have also rescued from their obscurity some of the classical early papers on the subject, which have been lost to sight and buried in the columns of out of date medical journals.

I realised when I began this work that a history written by an ex-anæsthetist who was prepared to devote unlimited time to it would be different from those already written. But I did not realise how different. The work meant such a surfeit of copying that, whenever possible, it aroused a strong desire to see things for myself. All the books record Hannah Greener's death under chloroform—the first anæsthetic fatality. But no one has gone to Winlaton and photographed the entry about her in the Register of Burials. No one has previously attempted to find out the extent of Syme's experience of chloroform at the time when he gave his dogmatic lecture on its absolute safety. This led to devastating numbers of deaths, and to the investigations of the Hyderabad and other chloroform Commissions. It was surprising to find out how small his experience really was, how utterly insufficient as a basis for his confident and cocksure statements. He claimed absolute safety after a mere two thousand cases! And, be it remembered, chloroform's worst enemies have never accused it of causing more than one death in a thousand, or even two thousand.

A clue which might have raised doubts about this omniscience earlier was the fact that he only devoted part of one lecture (about ten minutes) to the whole of anæsthesia, which shows how trivial his knowledge was compared to that of his contemporaries Snow and Clover.

In writing a preface I hesitated between two ideals. One was to say, "There is no preface. If the author can't make his meaning clear in several hundred pages he cannot improve matters by adding a few hundred extra words at the beginning." The other was to make a proper job of it and write a long one, which perhaps suits the plan of this book better. Most of the chapters themselves are essays only. I came across some point which interested me, burrowed like a ferret into my card index to get some more data, and then wrote an essay. To write a connected, consecutive history would be to repeat much that has already been written—and well written—by others. Also that way can lead to

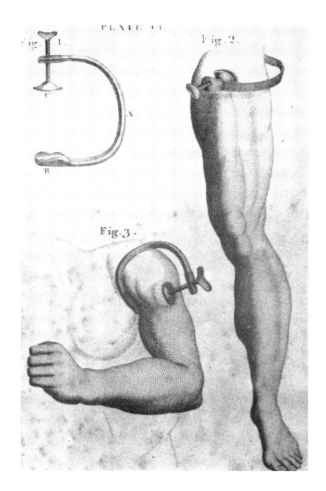

PLATE IX

System of Surgery. Benjamin Bell. 6th edition. 7 volumes. 1796. Vol. VII. Plate C1. Mr. James Moore of London suggested this nerve compressor to reduce pain during amputations. It must be used for one hour at least. It is made of curved iron covered with leather. This instrument is mentioned in many of the history books, but I have never before seen it illustrated. This book was one of the many borrowed from the Cambridge University Library.

facing page 14

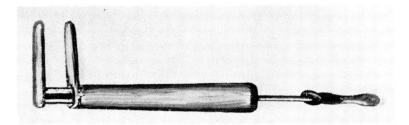

PLATE X

Lancet, 1916, June 24. 1249. A very early form of gag, long before the anæsthetic era. From *A System of Surgery,* by Benjamin Bell. Vol. 4. 1786. Quoted by W. H. Kelson. Recommended for amputation of the uvula.

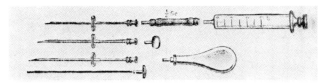

PLATE XI

Here is another good example of the re-invention of old ideas. Lemmon introduced continuous spinal anæsthesia in 1940. This "new" method was used thirty-three years earlier by Dean.

Brit. med. J., 1907, Oct. 5. 870. H. P. Dean. London Hospital. Spinal anæsthesia with stovaine. Made by Down Bros. "One can leave a needle in the canal during the operation, and at any moment some more drug can be injected without moving the patient."

monumental dullness and boredom. After all, in the words of Leonard Williams, why should medicine be dull as well as difficult? Very often the chase of something interesting led to a dead end—but the chase itself was interesting, even if it was not complete.

I have never seen or heard of a book with illustrations in the preface —which seems to me a very good reason why I should illustrate this one! For by now I have postponed my original idea, or rather modified it. The cost of thousands of illustrations would be large. No book of this kind can be a best seller, therefore no publisher can be expected to bear the risks himself. Even publishers have to live. That is the Law of Nature No. 1. The second Law of Nature is that, no matter how rich a person is, he is apt to turn a frosty eye upon a casual individual who drops in and tries to touch him for several thousand pounds for an enterprise that will interest only a limited number of people. I verified this second law experimentally on several occasions. Then I set my sights lower and decided to write an ordinary book, mostly print with a reasonable number of illustrations. This would be much cheaper to publish.

For sheer ingenuity the designs which appeal to me are the slow motion, automatic, hydrostatic syringe, and the two devices which blow a whistle when the gas cylinder is running out in the darkness of the X-ray room.

For charm I give first place to the little man in the bowler hat (Derby hat, I believe, in America), who is manfully turning a large wheel by hand to compress oxygen into cylinders in the early years of the century. He probably, at that date, got as much as sixteen or seventeen shillings a week for this labour of Hercules. That would be $4 to $4.25. I almost think I should have taken off my bowler hat for this job.

A fact which surprised me was the number of transfusion apparatuses designed by intrepid individuals who knew nothing and cared less about the mysteries of blood grouping or even asepsis, which lay hidden in the future. They begin as early as 1858, whereas Lister did not begin to teach surgeons to be clean until 1867, and there was a spate of them during the eighties, although blood grouping was not known at all until 1900.

For pathos my sympathies are entirely with Clover in his valiant efforts to give gas to heavily bearded gentlemen who must have leaked air from every point of the compass.

I am afraid the booby prize for design must be given to no less a man than Lawson Tait. He was a brilliant surgeon, a fearless pioneer in abdominal work, in which he had considerable success, despite his scorn

One of the purposes of my proposed complete pictorial encyclopædia was that you could find out from it how many times your new ideas had been used before. Here is a good example.

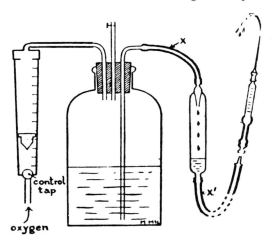

FIG. 9

Lancet, 1940, Nov. 23, 650. R. R. Macintosh and E. A. Pask. Continuous intravenous apparatus. Steady pressure from an oxygen cylinder fitted with a reducing valve forces the liquid out of the bottle. The middle tube can be used to reduce or release the pressure. The weak point of this apparatus is that the bottle must not be allowed to get empty, or disastrous gas embolism will occur. To avoid this the same authors brought out an improved model about seven months later.

FIG. 10

Lancet, 1941, July 5. 10. In this, as long as there is fluid in the dropper chamber the float is lifted away from its seat and the fluid can flow into the veins. But if the fluid is exhausted the float drops and fits into a ground seating at the bottom of the chamber and cuts off the air flow. The dropper chamber is made of Pyrex glass.

FIG. 11

This was a great improvement, but it was not new.
Medical Times and Gazette, 1866, Aug. 4. 113. B. W. Richardson described his apparatus for intravenous injection. This was designed for use in a cholera epidemic, which was then prevalent. He suggested a mixture of white of egg, salt, carbonate of soda, animal fat, glycerine and water. It is included here for comparison with Macintosh and Pask's apparatus of 75 years later. The principle of the automatic safety stop valve is identical.

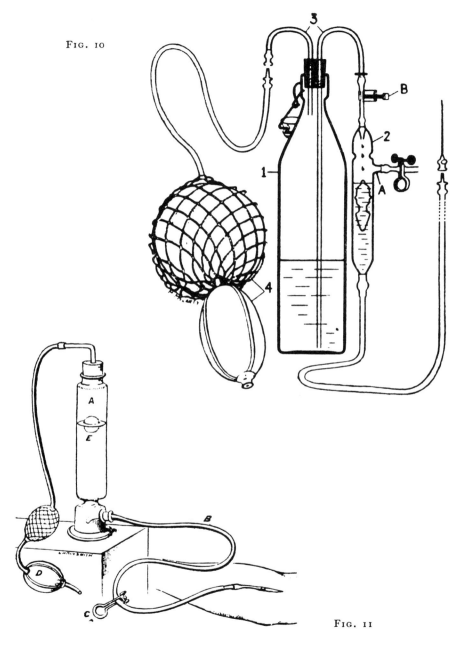

Fig. 10

Fig. 11

of Lister's methods, and above all, a merciless, truculent and pugnacious controversialist. You have only to look at his face to see what an auto-cratic, dictatorial slave-driver he was—though he probably drove himself harder than anyone else. As a designer of anæsthetic apparatus, however, he cannot be allotted many marks. He actually produced a glass vessel in which ether was heated by the naked flame of a spirit lamp! I should imagine that he only used it once, and that for a very short time. At any rate, there is no further mention of it in history.

Mr. Leslie's armchair was chosen for this preface out of about fifty illustrations of different methods of artificial respiration. It stands out above all others, *hors concours*, as the most stupid machine ever designed. The only thing to be said in its favour is that, unlike Lawson Tait's inhaler, it won't blow up or burst into flames.

Corning's spinal needle was selected for its very advanced design; the gag for its antiquity; the air raid syringe as a comment on modern civilisation. The continuous intravenous apparatus and the continuous spinal method are shown merely to illustrate the frequency with which things are re-invented.

GLENHOLME,
   MORLEY,
      LEEDS. 1960.

W. STANLEY SYKES.

CONTENTS

PLATES

ILLUSTRATIONS

CHAPTER I

INTRODUCTORY

THE EFFECT OF CANTHARIDES ON THE HEDGEHOG

"Is there any other point to which you would wish to draw my attention?"
"To the curious incident of the dog in the night-time."
"The dog did nothing in the night-time."
"That was the curious incident," remarked Sherlock Holmes.

—Sir ARTHUR CONAN DOYLE, *Silver Blaze*.

THE passage of forty-five years has wiped from my memory much detail which cost a lot of labour to acquire when I was a medical student. But in many of the varied subjects which we studied there was one absurd fact of such outstanding futility that it was utterly and completely unforgettable. The passage of the years makes no difference to it. Nothing will ever erase it.

No one, for example, could possibly fail to remember the anatomical detail that the nerve to the teres minor has a gangliform enlargement upon it. Years after I had forgotten the nerve supply to the teres minor —even the very whereabouts of that obscure and unimportant muscle— I remember its gangliform enlargement, which is of absolutely no significance at all to anybody. It is not even a proper ganglion. If it had been I should have forgotten it long since.

In pharmacology most of the things I learned are now completely obsolete, and are not even mentioned in modern text-books. But one pharmacological fact remains with me to this day, which will never be out-dated, which will always be remembered. Far from being obsolete it has assumed a greater importance than ever before—and that is the classically inane statement that cantharides has no effect upon the hedgehog. Unforgettable? Yes. Asinine and imbecile? Not altogether.

Now cantharides is a drug which is practically never used, and very few people are interested in the love life of hedgehogs, except perhaps to wonder vaguely whether it must not be somewhat difficult at the best of times. But the point of this ridiculous statement is—and it is apt to be forgotten by the increasing number of people whose whole life is bounded by laboratory walls—that it is highly dangerous and misleading to transfer the results of animal experiments to human beings, or even to other species of animals. For if cantharides has no effect on the hedgehog it has a very definite and sometimes disastrous effect upon humans.

The rabbit, I believe, is immune to belladonna and can eat the plant with impunity, but this does not mean that children can do the same. A small dog can take a grain of morphia hypodermically as a therapeutic dose—that is normal veterinary practice—but a man of eight times the dog's weight would not react at all well to a dose of eight grains.

Knowledge may be gained in at least three different ways. There is the experimental or inductive method, which reasons from particular instances to general principles; this has had a very good innings for the last three hundred years, and especially for the last hundred. On it is founded the enormous prestige and colossal achievements of modern science. It is an excellent method which produces results in plenty, and reliable results so long as we do not transfer the findings of experiments to surroundings in which they no longer apply. In other words, so long as we don't dose the baby with cantharides, relying on its harmlessness to the hedgehog.

Then there is the deductive method in which results are deduced by pure logic from accepted principles or premises. This method is often thought to be out-dated, to be a sterile and mediæval pursuit which leads nowhere. But it is not a bad method, so long as the premises from which you argue are correct. If they are not, the strictest rules of logic will not keep you out of trouble. But this is not a fault of the method itself—it is merely that the method is badly applied. If the foundation stones are crooked no levels and no set squares will ensure the stability of the building which rests on them.

For example the chloroform enthusiasts argued that it was not possible to get drunk on too little whisky, which seems on the face of it to be absolutely sound commonsense and utterly incontrovertible. But they then transferred this argument to chloroform, and stoutly maintained that it was not possible to have a death in light and early anæsthesia, quite regardless of the fact that deaths under these very conditions were occurring every week. The columns of the nineteenth century journals abound with them.

What the enthusiasts failed to allow for was the effect of fear and its accompanying hyperadrenalinæmia, which were later found to be the exact conditions required to cause sudden death under light chloroform anæsthesia. They argued quite correctly from their premises, but the premises were not accurate. The problem was assumed to be simple light anæsthesia, whereas it was in reality light anæsthesia plus an autogenous drug produced by fear.

Then there is the historical method of acquiring knowledge, which can often correct the faults of the other methods—inaccurate observations or ill-chosen premises. History is often unthinkingly dismissed as inter-

24

esting—or uninteresting, as the case may be—but of no practical importance. Why should an anæsthetist, for example, know anything about the history of his subject, except as a matter of academic interest? Is he any the better for knowing it?

Yes, he is, for it is one of the branches of research, and without research of some kind the anæsthetist is a mere technician. I gave up anæsthetics, the one great interest of my life, because the conditions under which I worked for over twenty years made me a technician and nothing more. An experience of sixteen thousand anæsthetics hammered something into me, but it was not enough. I was learning very little, and the penalty for not learning could occasionally be death—for somebody else. So I gave it up—it was just as simple as that. (The coming of the National Health Service has altered things to the extent that nowadays anybody in this country who is really keen on anæsthetics can make a living out of it).

The history of anæsthesia abounds with lethal devices and dangerous methods which were revived and re-introduced time after time by people who did not know that they had been tried before and given up because they were too lethal. It was not an anæsthetist, I am glad to say, who introduced chloroform capsules for use by unsupervised midwives, as though the most dangerous drug of all, which had been almost abandoned by skilled anæsthetists all over the world, could be safely revived, in any form or in any dosage, for use by the unskilled.

Records and statistics also form part of the historical method, and they are becoming more and more important with the increasing number of new and different methods tried out. It has come to be recognised that it is not enough to talk airily about "many hundreds of cases," or "thirty or forty thousand cases," both of which phrases were used by nineteenth century writers. It is a slow method and it has the disadvantage that statistics will never give results applicable to the individual. But a slow advance is better than no advance at all, and a method found to be safe in mass experiments will usually also be safe for any individual in that mass.

There may also be other ways of gaining knowledge—most unlikely ways. All things are possible in a world where a study of serial sections of mosquitos' stomachs was directly responsible for the successful building of the world's mightiest canal.

CHAPTER 2

THE ENVIRONMENT OF ANÆSTHESIA;
ITS VICTORIAN AGE BACKGROUND

WHAT sort of society was it at the time when the news of anæsthesia arrived from America? What were the living conditions of the doctors of England—and their patients?

It was a crude and brutal age for the majority of people, tempered only by extreme privileges reserved strictly for the favoured few. Lord Cardigan, who led the charge of the Light Brigade at Balaclava in 1854—an incident which, on a smaller scale, equalled Pickett's charge at Gettysburg nine years later in its reckless heroism—lived in comfort on board his private yacht whilst his men starved and froze on shore. It was an age when public executions were regarded as a form of entertainment.

Bendigo was champion of England's prize-ring for the second time—for America's monopoly of the heavyweight championship had not yet begun. It is true that Thomas Molyneaux, the negro slave from Virginia, had made the attempt many years before, in 1810, but the result had not encouraged other Americans to follow his example. For he had Tom Cribb, the reigning champion, helplessly beaten at the beginning of the twenty-fourth round. Cribb's second then made a false accusation that the negro had concealed stones in his hands, and the resulting wrangle to disprove this gained a vital extra minute's rest for Cribb, who went on to win in the thirty-fourth round. The champion himself had nothing to do with this, but the sharp practice of his second, and of the referee who allowed it to pass, left a very nasty smell behind it.

The working classes had an extremely raw deal. Wages were very poor indeed, even allowing for the low cost of living in those days. Only by working atrociously long hours, generally under vile conditions, could a workman make enough to support his family at a very low standard of living. Nothing was left over for the payment of such luxuries as doctors' bills.

Even as late as 1908[1] a trouser finisher was paid 2/- per dozen pairs, which meant that she earned 1¾d. an hour, or ten shillings for five working days of thirteen hours—and she had to find her own machine and thread.

Match box makers were paid 2d. a gross, which gave them 7/- for a fifty-two hour week. A blouse maker was even worse paid at 1d. an hour.

In 1846 Mr. Wakley, the energetic and formidable editor of *The Lancet*, presented a petition to the House of Commons asking for a Bill to prohibit all persons under 21 from being worked in factories for more than ten hours a day. This was a lot worse than it sounds, for "under twenty-one" meant, in many cases, children of six years old.

In 1840 appeared the first postage stamp—the famous penny black of Queen Victoria. As it was the only one in the world at the time there was no need to label it with its country of origin. To this day British stamps, with sublime but historical insolence, still do not insert the name of the country—the only ones in the world which do not.

In 1847 *The Lancet* protested against the Army practice of branding deserters with the letter D, saying with considerable commonsense that the best way to prevent desertion was to make the service desirable. A War Office order directed that the branding should be carried out under the superintendence of Army surgeons, which aroused *The Lancet's* indignation. "This association of the Army surgeons with the duties of the provost-marshal is most disgraceful to the military profession and degrading to its medical officers."

But even worse than this took place. After all, the act of branding, painful, degrading and unnecessary as it may have been, was quickly over and involved no risk to life. It had, in fact, the advantage that it was the one and only operation performed at that time with a sterile instrument. It is quite literally true to say that branding by the heavy hands of the regimental farrier was less risky than a minor operation carried out by one of the acknowledged surgical masters such as Syme or Astley Cooper.

Flogging was a different matter altogether. It was nothing less than prolonged torture with a very definite risk to life. In June, 1846, a young soldier of the 7th Hussars, Private F. J. White, aged 27, assaulted a sergeant.[2] After trial and sentence by a District Court Martial he received 150 lashes on the 15th June. And this was a very moderate number by the standards of the time. Five hundred lashes were fairly common and a thousand not unknown. Private White died in hospital on 11th July, and the inquest lasted four days. *The Lancet* devoted fourteen columns to it, in very small print, about ten thousand words, and so gave a very full account of a case which nearly escaped publicity altogether.

Mr. Wakley, the Editor, happened also to be the Coroner, and once the matter was reported to him, he had not the least intention of allowing it to be hushed up. He investigated the details carefully and thoroughly and many damaging facts emerged. The regimental surgeon, Dr. Warren, was present at the flogging, but did not examine the man at the time, nor did he see him again until ten o'clock the next morning. By that time the patient had had no food for seventeen hours. A Staff-surgeon Hall was sent to see him by the Director General of the Army Medical Department just before he died. Three Army doctors did the post-mortem and found "marks of corporal punishment across the shoulders, particularly over the right scapula; but the punishment does not appear to have been severe, and the part where it was inflicted is quite healed."

A flogging followed by twenty-six days in hospital and death at the end of it "does not appear to have been severe"! The obvious question is, what would have been the effect of a severe flogging? Mr. Wakley was obviously thinking along these lines, for he settled down to a long and patient investigation. A certificate had been given that "death was in no wise connected with corporal punishment," on the grounds that a pleural effusion was present. Private White had apparently died of pure cussedness, or perhaps of malingering. The white-washing process had begun, but it was very soon checked, in the first place at the instance of the local Vicar. The death was registered in the ordinary way, but the Vicar had heard about the flogging, and to his credit he refused to carry out the burial until he had notified the coroner. Then the balloon went up.

Mr. Wakley had no use for the white-wash brush, and very soon discovered that only the skin of the back had been removed at the post-mortem, and that, although the parts under it had been stated to be sound and undamaged, they had only been superficially inspected. He asked the jury to have an independent examination carried out. Mr. Day, a surgeon, repeated the post-mortem, but he, in his turn did not examine any more closely. The reason for this extraordinary omission is not stated. Mr. Day must surely have known the reason for his re-examination. Anyway, the coroner refused to hear his evidence, and no doubt refused to pay his fee. Then it was the jury's turn to ask Mr. Wakley to nominate an independent examiner. Erasmus Wilson, one of the earliest derma-tologists, was commissioned to carry out yet another examination, and he found that the deep muscles of the back were ecchymosed and pulpy, and swore that the underlying disease (pleural effusion) was related to this—that in fact the flogging was the cause of death.

The jury returned a verdict to this effect, and added that "they could not restrain from expressing their horror and disgust at . . . the law of this realm which permits this revolting punishment to be inflicted upon British soldiers, and . . . implored every man in the Kingdom to join . . . in forwarding petitions to the Legislature, praying in the most urgent terms, for abolition of every law, order and regulation, which permits flogging to remain one moment longer a slur upon the humanity and fair name of the people of this country."

This did not have much immediate effect. Flogging was not abolished in the Army until 1881—thirty-five years after this case.

Mr. Wakley's behaviour was later criticised in Parliament, but he had wisely taken the precaution of obtaining letters from the Vicar, the solicitor who represented the officers concerned and from a barrister, who all spoke very highly of the unbiassed and patient care with which the enquiry had been undertaken. So the coroner-editor was in an impregnable position. Mr. Wakley had had an extensive experience of rows of all kinds—ten libel actions in ten years stood to his credit—for he was an indefatigable smeller-out of scandals, and he had nothing to learn about protecting himself from retaliation.

Modern medical journals are of a very high standard, and are sometimes a trifle dull in their frigid respectability and their scientific outlook. No ripple of sensationalism ever disturbs the serene surface of their columns. It was not always so, especially with Mr. Wakley. In 1838 the usual students' number appeared at the beginning of the academic year, and the editor reviewed for his readers the staffs of the teaching hospitals.

"Mr. White, as he himself knows, is an exceedingly clever man, and as all the world knows, a very lazy one." This is the rapier thrust which the editor aims at one surgeon. The next on the list is treated far more roughly. "Of Sir Anthony Carlisle we need only say that he is in a state of *delirium tremens*." The unfortunate baronet thus bludgeoned was an ex-President of the College of Surgeons and senior surgeon at one of the famous London hospitals. A month or two later Sir Anthony made a rather careless mistake in a lunacy certificate, whereupon the watchful editor descends upon him once again. "The reckless folly of an antiquated surgical Merry-Andrew" is merely a prelude to the following astounding indictment: "He is not only incapable of performing any capital operation but even any ordinary operation, without danger to his patient. He is not only incompetent, but he has been so for the last ten years, and his daily increasing imbecility and senility render him more and more useless."

This amazing editor was absolutely without fear. Rank, position and power counted for nothing in his eyes, and this at a time when rank and position were almost all-powerful; and the more exalted his opponent the more joyously he entered the fray. The next victim was no less a person than Sir Henry Halford, President of the Royal College of Physicians. This gentleman, accompanied by a friend, was on his way to a dinner appointment. The friend was striken by a hemiplegia in the train, whereupon Sir Henry left him at a wayside station and went on to the dinner. Mr. Wakley devotes several editorials to the careful and conscientious scarification of Sir Henry.

"If neither friendship nor kindness could have swayed this physician to . . . his duty, a regard for consistency should have had that effect. Upon all occasions . . . he has obtruded his religious creed and feelings upon the . . . public. He has done this in the most offensive manner."

Was the law of libel weak in those days, or was it merely the normal brutality of an age which operated without anæsthetics? In any case it made *The Lancet* highly stimulating and entertaining reading.

In the next year after the flogging incident another case aroused Mr. Wakley's wrath. Mary Ann Hunt was charged with murder at the Central Criminal Court and found guilty. She pleaded pregnancy, and a jury of twelve matrons was sworn. Mr. Baron Platt, the Judge, told them that they were at liberty to have the assistance of a surgeon if they thought it necessary. But the jury of matrons took it upon themselves to say she was not pregnant, whereupon the judge directed that the law must take its course.

The Lancet pointed out that in similar cases, when the jury of matrons had given their verdict, living children had sometimes been born in the interval between the verdict and the execution. Why was not the jury directed to obtain a proper obstetric opinion, instead of being told that they *might* call in a surgeon?

Mr. Wakley was talking sense, for it happened again in this very case. The sentence was passed in September and Mrs. Hunt gave birth to a child in December. Three doctors, by order of the Home Secretary, had examined her by early October and found her to be pregnant.

At this time the large hospitals each had one regular operating session per week. It was all that was needed. In 1846 one of the attractions of Glasgow as a centre for medical students was the fact that the total number of operations was 120 annually. This enormous total of two every week apparently applied to the united work of three hospitals!

Nor were the hospitals themselves exactly havens of peace and tranquility. *The Lancet* has some very acid comments to make on the Board of the Westminster Hospital,[3] which one would expect to be a dignified and austere body, with all the primness of Victorian respectability.

"At the weekly Board, held on Wednesday last, a most disgraceful *rencontre* took place before the governors of this ancient and excellent institution. Mr. Guthrie, formerly surgeon to the hospital, and late President of the Royal College of Surgeons, actually threatened to throw Dr. Kingston, one of the physicians of the institution, out of the boardroom window. If such scenes as these are to be the result of Mr. Guthrie's reappearances in the hospital, the sooner the governors interfere the better. The window from which Dr. Kingston was threatened to be hurled is about thirty feet from the ground!"

In 1847 the Students' Number appeared as usual at the beginning of the academic year. The Duke of Wellington, a crusted old Tory who opposed any change as a matter of principle, was Chancellor of the University of Oxford. Cambridge was more fortunate in having the progressive and very intelligent Prince Albert as its titular head.

The Royal College of Physicians of London still called upon their examination candidates to translate into Latin a passage from Hippocrates, Galen or Aretæus.

In 1860 Mr. McDougall[4] leased the sewage of Carlisle and 100 acres of land. He treated the sewage with carbolic acid solution at a cost of 5/3 per day or £95 a year. He found that this made the sewage inoffensive and his 100 acres were transformed into valuable farmland. This was the experiment which decided Lister, a few years later, to use carbolic acid in order to put the coping stone of antiseptic surgery on to Pasteur's researches on fermentation.

In 1897 another hint of modern times appears. "The motor car has taken its first toll of human life in London, a child, aged nine years, having lost his life through the agency of one in Hackney, on Sept. 22nd."

Three years later[5] *The Lancet* commented upon a temperance drink which had recently become popular as a teetotal substitute for brandy. It was composed of equal parts of strong tincture of ginger, sal volatile and chloric ether. *The Lancet* pointed out that whereas brandy contained 50% of alcohol by volume, its teetotal substitute contained no less than 83%! No wonder it was popular, for it contained the kick of a mule with the pleasing consciousness of virtue!

Another three years later, though this fell just outside the Victorian era, a nostalgic advertisement appeared in the *Medical Annual*.[6] A special whisky was advertised for diabetics, and being specially prepared, it was much more expensive than ordinary brands. Forty-nine shillings—about what one pays today for a bottle of special whisky—but the forty-nine shillings was the price of a dozen bottles! A single bottle cost 4/1 or 98 cents, ordinary whisky was 3/6 or 84 cents.

A glimpse of late nineteenth century general practice can be obtained from "A digest of a midwifery notebook."[7] This interested me particularly because it happens to refer to the small town in which I live. Dr. West, who wrote the article, I can faintly remember. The doctor whose note-book he used died three years before I was born, but I have heard his name mentioned by patients many times.

From 1858 until his death in 1891, a period of 33 years, Charles Hirst, L.R.C.P., L.S.A., practised medicine in Morley, Yorkshire. 8,629 confinements are noted in his books, of which he personally attended 46% (over 3,960). His greatest number in one year was 462. He had 15 mater-nal deaths in all. Only 13 occipito-posterior positions occurred, which seems an unusually small proportion. His operative deliveries included vectis 2, craniotomy 8, decapitation 1, forceps 148 (1·7%, or 3·7% if the lower figure be taken.)

Ether was given in one case only and chloroform in one, so he was not an enthusiastic anæsthetist. Placenta prævia occurred 13 times and post-partum hæmorrhage 62 times.

The two total figures are a little confusing. Probably they mean that he was "booked" for the 8,629, but owing to their vast numbers and the pressure of his other work he was only present at the actual delivery in the 3,960.

Even allowing for the fact that the birth rate then was very much higher than it is now, and for the fact that there were no certificated midwives and no maternity homes then, which deal with the majority of confinements today, the numbers are astonishing.

What a terrible, galley-slave life he must have led. An unbroken night's sleep must have been almost unknown, and his daily work, apart from midwifery, must have been enormous, for the number of his obstetric cases implies a very large practice. Moreover he had to walk to his cases, or perhaps for the more distant ones ride a bicycle or saddle a horse in the middle of the night, with all that these implied in exposure to rain, snow and wind. Not for him was the luxury of an easily started car with good weather protection. Nor for him was the convenience of electric light, constant hot water or other comforts. Nor could he put on comfortable and informal clothes, even in the night, such as the navy duffle coat and the air force flying boots which are two of the good things to come out of the war. The ironclad, inflexible rule then was that a top hat and frock coat must be worn on all occasions and at all times, whatever, the weather and whatever the patient's status.

His maximum ordinary fee for a confinement would be one guinea, very often not paid, or half a guinea if it was a pauper case, paid for by the Guardians.

No wonder that he was only present at the actual birth in less than half the cases. It was physically impossible to do more.

The style in which the nineteenth century journals were written is apt to be somewhat irritating—it is so verbose and long-winded. It completely lacked the sonorous beauty of Elizabethan prose and the workmanlike brevity of (some) modern literature, and the only effect it achieved was that of unimpressive pomposity. No one ever used a short sentence if it could be made into a long one with plenty of commas. The simple verb "I think" was never used. It was always "I cannot but think."

Dr. C. D. Arnott (not to be confused with James Arnott, one of the pioneers of freezing for local anæsthesia) in describing obsterical analgesia, says, "a lawn handkerchief was moistened with half a drachm of the fluid, and was held over the mouth and nose a short time antecedent to the accession of the uterine throes." Translated, this means simply, before each pain.

All letters to the editor began, "I crave your indulgence for trespassing upon your valuable space," or "I cannot but think it ought to be recorded, and venture to hope that you may find room for it in your next issue." Quite a lot of valuable space could have been saved and a great deal more room found, if they hadn't talked about it so much.

In 1829 one gentleman took up a whole page of 1,500 words to describe a flexible stethoscope.

"Sir,—It having been suggested to me, that notice of a modified stethoscope, which has been successfully used in the Royal Infirmary, Edinburgh, would perhaps meet your eye from another pen, if mine were not employed, I beg leave to trouble you with a description of the following instrument. I should not, however, have had the hardihood to obtrude this letter upon your notice, had not others beside myself been experimentally satisfied of the truth of the details herein made. If this paper should appear not unworthy of mention, I shall send a drawing of the instrument, with a report of its effects, and the result of an experiment respecting the condensation of the air in the stethoscope during exploration. . . ."

Having occupied all this space in saying precisely nothing at all, it can be imagined how he spread himself when it came to describing the instrument, with the result that there wasn't room for the drawing after all.

Another contributor referred to "concomitant affections of the nose and throat which require synchronous treatment." All he meant was adenoids.

Referring to the chewing of tobacco in hospital wards (needless to add it was always called the fragrant weed), an anti-tobacconist whose grammar is more shaky than his opinions writes: "such a disgusting practice being obvious incompatible of that state of cleanliness that should obtain in all nosocomial establishments." Apart from the sheer gobbledegookery of it, it is difficult to imagine that even spitting on the floor would make any difference to the septic horrors of hospitals at that time! Sawdust on the floor of the operating theatre, knives stropped on the boot and held in the surgeon's mouth until wanted and ligatures knotted in the buttonhole of an old and dirty frock coat—what did it matter if the chewer missed the spittoon?

The economics of general practice in the nineteenth century make depressing reading. In 1847 Dr. F. S. Garlick, one of the medical officers to the Halifax Poor Law Guardians, gives some details of the payment he received for the treatment of paupers, that derogatory word applied to all who needed poor law assistance. His salary was £80 a year, or 4/4½d. a day, or one dollar and five cents at the then fixed rate of exchange (this was one of the good things of the Victorian age. For with the massive commonsense which distinguished them, in some respects at least, the Victorians did not, as we do today, measure the value of things with an elastic foot rule.)

He gives a list of the work done in thirty-one days during May and June. The salary for the period was £6. 15. 7½d. (33 dollars 87 cents). For that he paid 427 visits, supplied 447 mixtures, 992 pills, 254 powders, 17 lotions, 2 liniments, 25 ointments and 32 plasters. This makes his gross remuneration 3¾d. (7½ cents) per visit, which includes supplying all the above mentioned drugs. Any profit remaining was entirely his own, for taxation was negligible in those days. Later the same year he gives further figures, for thirteen weeks this time. He received £20 salary for this quarter year, and made more profit, or rather a smaller loss, for he received as much as sevenpence a visit during this period. He listed 685 visits, 985 mixtures, 2,255 pills and 879 powders.

Emboldened by his example, Dr. T. Harrison, medical officer to another of the Halifax districts, sent in some statistics of his own. In one week he did 44 visits with a mileage of 40 miles, including the usual vast supplies of medicine, for a total salary of 9/9½d, an average rate of just over 2½d. per visit.

Dr. H. B. Davies of Llanerchymedd, was at first sight more fortunate or more generously paid. His £60 a year salary paid him almost a shilling a visit, but at the cost of travelling nearly two thousand miles a year. Two thousand miles, on foot or on horseback, was a long way and took up a lot of time—at the very least 500 hours, or 62 eight hour days.

Mr. Haslam, of Carnarvon, calculated his payment in a rather different way. He received £50 a year, but it cost him £40 in expenses —drugs, etc. This left him £10 a year, or 6½d. per day, for medical attendance on 2,600 persons. Whichever way you look at it the payment was fantastically bad.

There were other disadvantages about poor law work as well as the wretched pay. In 1847 three of the seventeen parish doctors in Glasgow died of fever, and three more of them were ill with it. They had received, according to *The Lancet's* calculations, three farthings (1½ cents) a visit for their work during an epidemic, presumably with the usual proviso that they had to supply medicines free out of their excess profits. *The Lancet* pointed out that nothing would be done unless medical men united to refuse the work, except at a proper salary. And in effect very little was done. No real improvement took place until well on into the twentieth century, when the old poor law was abolished altogether, regretted by nobody. Many other examples of the meanness of the guardians could be given. As even the authorities realised that the usual contract salaries were hardly generous, a scale of extra payments was laid down for certain specified operations or treatments which meant extra work for the doctor. But the guardians were not above dodging these payments if they possibly could, in their anxiety to save the ratepayers money. Quite a common procedure was to refuse payment for treatment for a dislocation or a fracture because the injury had been treated before a special order was obtained from the relieving officer, who might live many miles away, and who was in any case somewhat difficult of access for a patient with a broken leg. In another instance a reduction of a dislocated shoulder was refused payment because the printed scale said dislocation of the arm, and it was argued that a shoulder was not an arm.

One doctor received an order, duly signed, to visit a case of puerperal fever late at night. The patient lived three miles away, and daily visits were paid for a week, sometimes twice a day. So at the very least eight visits were paid, which involved 48 miles travelling, which would take 12 hours or more. The doctor applied for a modest fee of £1, and was refused. He appealed to the Commissioners, feeling that he was on safe ground, having a relieving officer's order. But they also refused to pay, stating that puerperal fever on the eleventh day is not a confinement.

In the nineteenth century poverty was regarded as a crime and treated as such, but the poor were kept poor by low wages which did not allow for any surplus or saving. When a person became unfit through illness, accident or old age, to earn even a small wage there was nothing left but starvation or the workhouse, a place regarded by the poor as a horror and a disgrace.

Not without reason, apparently. On May 20th, 1848, *The Lancet* had a leading article about the Huddersfield Workhouse.

"Patients have been allowed to remain for nine weeks together without a change of linen or bedclothing; beds in which patients suffering in typhus have died, one after the other, have been again and again and repeatedly used for fresh patients, without any change or attempt at purification; the said beds were only bags of straw or shavings, for the most part laid on the floor, and the whole swarmed with lice; two patients suffering in infectious fever were almost constantly put together in one bed; it not infrequently happened that one would be ragingly delirious, while the other was dying; and it is a fact that a living patient has occupied the same bed with a corpse for a considerable period after death; the patients have been for months together without proper appointed nurses to attend to them; there has been for a considerable time none but male paupers to attend on female patients; when the poor creatures were laid in the most abject and helpless state—so debilitated as to pass their ejections as they lay—they have been suffered to remain in the most befouled state possible, besmeared in their own excrement for days together and not even washed."

This was an indictment put forward by a responsible journal. I think it must be accepted as true, at the time. It must be remembered that workhouses have long since disappeared from the face of this realm. Another point to remember is that when *The Lancet* criticises the absence of nurses—what it really means is the absence of attendants, for this was the pre-Nightingale era, and there were no such things as nurses, educated to be such. The Prince Consort himself, during his fatal attack of typhoid fever, a disease in which skilled nursing was of the utmost importance, didn't get it because it did not exist.

But is it any wonder that workhouses were not popular? Traces of the same attitude lingered on into the twentieth century right up to the 1914 war, which was the real end of the nineteenth century, so we need not feel too self-righteous. As late as 1909 *The Lancet* reported the Salford Guardians' "amazing request" that brushes and combs be provided for infirmary patients. Evidently some of the Guardians were moving with the times. But at another Board meeting there was "derisive laughter" when it was proposed to provide workhouse children with toothbrushes. Mental hospitals were not much better.[8]

"At the Asylum of West Auckland, first visited on the 5th of Dec., 1842. . . . In the small, cheerless dayroom of the males, with only one unglazed window, five men were restrained by leg-locks, called hobbles, and two were wearing, in addition, iron handcuffs, and fetters from the wrist to the ankle; they were all tranquil. . . . One woman was leg-locked by day and chained to her bed at night; chains were fastened to the floors in many places, and to many of the bedsteads. The males . . . slept two in one bed. I have seen one secured in a dark and loathsome shed, lying extended upon straw (for the space did not admit of his standing erect), in a state of filth that I dare not describe; a second was fettered and manacled, and basking in the public street, exposed to the rude gaze of the thoughtless passersby; a third I have seen led about the streets, and even to church, in the restraint of a strait-waiscoat; a fourth . . . died some time ago . . . having been for about fifteen years chained."

Nor did emigrants fare any more luxuriously.[9]

"Five hundred poor ignorant creatures, of both sexes and of all ages . . . are huddled and crowded into this place (the 'tween decks). . . . The normal contract is that the ship is to supply fuel and water, but the passengers . . . provide their own food. . . . The means provided for cooking are on deck . . . (and) totally useless in bad weather. The ship has scarcely left her port of departure before every passenger is down with sea sickness. When night approaches the hatches are closed. The air below soon becomes pestiferous . . ."

The rise of some of the special departments was also slow and painful.[10] James Berry related an incident which he had seen himself. When gynæcologists were only beginning to operate he saw an elderly gynæcologist (trained as a physician) struggling to remove a retro-peritoneal tumour. He asked Berry what it was. "One glance sufficed to show that it was a solitary, horseshoe kidney, which no one with any training in anatomy and pathology could have failed to recognise." He had already cut both ureters and the vessels, as revealed at the post-mortem the next day.

Club contracts were another very poorly paid part of general practice at that time, and they were very widespread in all parts of the country. Because the average workman simply could not afford to pay doctors' bills, modest as they were, the usual way out of the dilemma was to join a club, which collected a small weekly sum of a penny or two, or even less. The club then asked for contract tenders from the local doctors—so many hundred, or thousand, patients to be treated and supplied with medicine at a fixed rate per annum. The value of the rate per head was never high and usually very low. Three shillings a year, or less than a penny a week, was a common figure.

New comers or doctors with small practices and growing families tended to undercut their better established colleagues when tendering, in their anxiety to be sure of at least some certain income, no matter how small. Besides, a club practice might lead to an extension of the candidate's private practice.

A doctor in 1896, in a district of 6,000 people, had a practice almost entirely composed of club patients. The capitation fee was 3/- a year for adults, or ½d. a week for children, which could only yield 2/2 a year if nothing was charged for collection. And quite certainly an appreciable percentage would have to be deducted for this. The doctor probably got no more than 1/6 a year for children. But he could not complain or protest for fear of losing his livelihood. In this district even the richer people belonged to the clubs, including men who paid wages bills of £600 to £700 a week.

Assuming that this doctor had no competition whatever and that he had the whole population of 6,000 on his books, which is most unlikely, his earnings would be less than £700 a year, out of which he had to keep an assistant and three horses, for no man could even make a pretence of attending that number single-handed.

Why then did he not refuse to continue, if there was no opposition? Why did he not say, in future my capitation fee will be six shillings a year instead of three? The clubs had a very conclusive answer to that one. In the case of trouble they would simply persuade a newcomer to settle in the district by promising him a most rosy prospect, and perhaps even giving him a larger capitation fee—for a time—as a bait. Then the screw would be turned relentlessly. The newcomer's fees would be drastically cut, and if he didn't like it he could leave it. His former rival, who was probably starving by this time, would be only too pleased to get his clubs back again at any price.

Not that it cost very much to employ an assistant in those days. An advertisement in *The Times* in 1847 proves this: "A Gentleman, twenty-eight years of age, M.R.C.S. and L.A.C. (the usual double qualification then), wishes for a permanent situation as outdoor visiting or Dispensary Assistant to a respectable Practitioner, within a mile and a half of the Strand. Salary £50 per annum."

The Lancet comments that a gentleman's footman can get £40 per annum, with board, lodging and sometimes a suit or two of livery; but here we have an educated man proposing to toil, both mentally and physically, and that at all hours, for less remuneration than is accorded to a servant. Unqualified assistants, of course, came cheaper still, and were freely used. They were considered to be quite good enough for the poor, and there was no prohibition or restriction on their employment.

A letter from a military surgeon started another hare for Mr. Wakley in 1847. This doctor had returned from Canada on leave in one of H.M. ships and noticed that, while he messed in the wardroom, the Naval assistant surgeons were not allowed to mix with the other commissioned officers but messed with midshipmen, clerks and others of lowly rank. *The Lancet* commented acidly upon the status of these officers, pointing out that they slept in hammocks and had no cabin and no privacy of any sort. It was quite true that they were not allowed in the wardroom, which was open to second lieutenants of marines and Naval schoolmasters, who ranked below them.

The subject once being opened, there was a flood of complaints. One of these assistant surgeons describes his lot.[11] He was a qualified doctor after four years' apprenticeship and four years at the University. He had to mess in a filthy, dark den, called the midshipmen's berth, and associate solely with its occupants—a set of turbulent, half-educated schoolboys, whose "obscenities and blasphemies were truly horrible to any man of education.

"I was compelled to sleep in an open steerage, among a crowd of my noisy messmates, sailors and marines. . . . I was denied a cabin and a servant . . . there is a deep-rooted prejudice against us existing amongst all the executive officers, whose usual polite appellations for us are 'D——d civilians,' 'b——y sawbones,' etc. The merest boy of a naval cadet or clerk's assistant may address us in this disgusting language with perfect impunity. . . . Assistant surgeons in the Army, India Company, etc., whose qualifications are in no respect superior to ours, mess with field officers and captains of their respective regiments. Then why are we treated like boys—like menials?"

Promotion was very slow, so it was not as though the disadvantages applied for a short time only. Qualified men remained as assistant surgeons for as long as nine years, if they survived. In 1846 their full pay was seven shillings a day, rising after three years to seven and six and after ten years to nine shillings, a scale which obviously does not contemplate rapid advancement.

The very beginnings of the vast structure of modern public health and social welfare took place about the same time as the introduction of anæsthesia. Liverpool appointed Dr. Duncan in 1847 as the first Medical

Officer of Health in the country. The City of London followed suit the next year. Before this time the health of the public through sanitation, cleanliness and good working conditions was ignored completely. (This *laissez faire* attitude, while perhaps just tolerable when England was a rural country, produced most disastrous results when the Industrial Revolution crowded large masses of people into the towns and factories.

Charles Turner Thackrah (1795-1833), surgeon, of Leeds, was a general practitioner, but rather an unusual one. He ran a private school of anatomy and was thus indirectly one of the founders of the present University of Leeds. He also, in his spare time, founded the science of industrial medicine, by writing a book on the subject,[12] which makes grim reading.

Milliners and dressmakers, he says, "are often crowded in apartments of disproportionate size, and kept at work for an improper length of time. Their ordinary hours are ten to twelve a day, but they are confined not infrequently from five to six in the morning till twelve at night.

"Two very respectable dressmakers, who charge more than the generality, state that they can earn but 12s. (3 dollars) each per week, though they sew, on the average fifteen hours a day.

"Weavers by hand have low wages, and are often out of employ. Many an industrious man, working thirteen hours a day, earns no more than ten or twelve shillings a week. . . . In Spitalfields and Bethnal Green, where 1600 looms are at work, the silk weavers work at their own homes . . . when they have work they weave about sixteen hours a day, at the present (Sept. 1831) they can but earn nine shillings to eleven shillings per week."

Of power loom weaving—

"In one large establishment, in which were 70 male adults, we found 329 children, and 198 young women. . . . The labour commences at 6 in the morning, and ends at 7 in the evening; and allows intervals only of a quarter of an hour for breakfast, three quarters for dinner, and a quarter for 'drinking'. The hours are rigidly enforced in relation to all ages and classes of the operatives. In the employ, indeed, which requires attendance on machines no more time can be spared for rest, recreation or meals to the child 8 or 9 years old than to the adult.

"While the engine works, the people must work. Men, women and children, are thus yokefellows with iron and steam; the animal machine—fragile at best . . . is matched with an iron machine insensible to suffering or fatigue; all this, moreover, in an atmosphere of flax-dust, for 12 or 13 hours a day, and for six days in a week.

"Masons inhale particles of sand and dust, which arise from chipping the stone . . . masons are short-lived, dying generally before they attain the age of 40."

"The hours of labour (of colliers) are generally about 8 or ten daily. . . . Boys enter the pits at the age of six or seven, and are employed in opening the trap-doors, driving the horses, propelling the trucks, etc. . . . "

"Miners of lead suffer considerably from their employ . . . (they) rarely work more than six hours a day, yet they seldom attain the age of 40. They take immense quantities of ardent spirits . . . confessedly to drown the ever-recurring idea, that they are, from their occupation, doomed to premature disease. Last year, there were in the village of Arkendale (in the heart of the mining district), not less than thirty widows under thirty years of age."

"Fork-grinders, who use a dry grindstone, die at the age of 28 or 32, while the table knife grinders, who work on wet stones, survive to between 40 and 50."

"Persons commence the manufacture (of white lead) about the age of 20; many soon leave from broken health; those who endure the employ, do not remain on the average longer than the age of 45, and during one third of these 25 years, the men are laid up in bed, or decrepit from colic or palsy."

"I stood in Oxford-row, Manchester, and observed the streams of operatives as they left the mills, at 12 o'clock. The children were almost universally ill-looking, small, sickly, barefoot and ill-clad. Many appeared to be no older than seven. The men, generally from 16 to 24, and none aged, were almost as pallid and thin as the children. . . . Here I saw, or thought I saw, a degenerate race—human beings stunted, enfeebled, and depraved—men and women that were not to be aged—children that were never to be healthy adults."

But, before we part company with Mr. Thackrah, let us be fair. Unmercifully and relentlessly as the masters worked their men, they worked themselves just as hard. Speaking of one of them Mr. Thackrah says:

"He rises at five or soon after, and immediately enters the warehouse, which adjoins his house. At eight he steps home for breakfast, but returns again in fifteen or twenty minutes, and is at business till half-past one. He then goes to dinner, eats it hastily, rarely sits ten minutes afterwards, but proceeds to the warehouse. Tea and supper are uncertain, and one or the other is taken as convenient. The counting house is closed at nine or ten, and he remains with the clerks to the last."

These dreadful industrial conditions did not exist only in the early Victorian age. They persisted for more than fifty years after Mr. Thackrah's time. In 1883 *The Lancet* reported[13] that a woman making trousers earned one shilling a day, for which she worked seventeen hours —from 5 a.m. to 10 p.m. Shirt finishers get 3d. a dozen, out of which they had to buy their own thread. In 1888[14] girls carried half a hundredweight of moleskin trousers three miles home and received 4½d. a pair for making them up (and carrying them back again). This enabled them to earn from 2/6 to three shillings a week.

Work was carried on in filthy, overcrowded conditions, sometimes in cellars, sometimes in attics, with no available sanitation of any kind. One woman who worked from 8.30 a.m. to 7 p.m. for the magnificent sum of 2/2 a week (52 cents) had sixpence of this deducted because her employer supplied hot water for tea! No wonder shirts were advertised at three and sixpence each. Karl Marx certainly saw enough in Victorian England to start him on his career as a reformer. It is a pity that his dogmas, founded on conditions which have been utterly swept away, should have been raised to the rank of a religion.

Disraeli wrote a novel called *The Two Nations*, referring to the Victorian upper and lower classes. Two nations they were indeed, almost two species, and no doubt there was some foundation for the physical repulsion which the gentry felt for the working people at that time. They were, of necessity, badly dressed because they were very poor and new clothes never came their way. Second hand cast-offs were good enough for them. They were dirty and verminous because their work was dirty and they had no facilities for keeping themselves clean; they were illiterate because no schooling was provided and because they worked such long hours all through their childhood that they had neither the time nor the inclination to learn, much less time to play or time to live. Deformities due to bad food and bad working conditions, and skin diseases due to dirt were extremely common.

Dr. J. R. Lynch died during an epidemic of fever,[15] and *The Lancet* started a subscription for his wife and family. "In one small cellar," he said, "eighteen poor people lying on wet, dirty, straw. There was no window." In one house he counted eighty-one people, in another sixty-one, in every stage of fever, lying on straw in corners.

For these reasons the upper classes avoided any close contact with such sub-humans. What they did not realise was the fact that this dirty and verminous majority could in any way affect themselves at a distance. Secure, as they thought, in their wealth and the comforts and luxuries which accompanied it, they could not conceive that they were in any danger from the disease-ridden proletariat which they were helping to produce. So long as they did not mix and lived apart they could be ignored—that was the general opinion.

With poetic justice this ignorance exacted its own penalty. To mention only one example—and it must have happened many, many

33, The Folds,
Blackrod,
Bolton,
Gtr. Manchester

23rd April 1984

Dear Sir,

I wish to apply for the post of SHO in obstetrics

times—Queen Victoria herself, one of the great lovers of history, lost her beloved Albert for this very reason. She was powerful, rich, privileged, and had every known refinement of civilisation at her absolute disposal. No amount of trouble and no amount of expense needed to be spared in anything which concerned her and her family. Surely, above all other people, she was insulated from this particular danger.

Nevertheless the unfortunate Albert died in his prime from typhoid, a dirt disease. The magnificence of Windsor Castle and of the other royal palaces seemed to be a far cry from the dirty slums and the stinking cesspools of the poor, but they were near enough to be dangerous. Even the Castle battlements could not keep out the flies which came straight from the filth of the slums on to the royal table. That was in 1861. Ten years later H.R.H. the Prince of Wales (Edward VII) had a severe attack of typhoid, and twenty years later still, in 1891, Prince George of Wales (George V) also had it.

In 1885 *The Lancet* said, referring to the sanitary condition of Windsor,[16]

"the town is infected by a poisonous ditch . . . the inhabitants are still allowed to drink contaminated well-water . . . there are slums within a stone's throw of the Castle gates which are hotbeds of epidemic disease: and . . . even in the wealthiest quarters, complaints are constantly made of sewers that smell, and and open ditches which receive refuse, soil and the outflow from cesspools."

On the whole the Victorian era saw a tremendous change in medical science. It covered the birth of modern chemistry, the beginnings of public health and sanitation, though only the beginnings, the rise of bacteriology and the discovery of X-rays and the development of all other modern diagnostic methods and instruments.

The first news about "photography through opaque screens" occurs in January, 1896.[17] In the next issue of *The Lancet* the first X-ray photograph was published. It showed the bones of a hand, with an exposure of $4\frac{1}{2}$ minutes.

The two most spectacular discoveries were those of anæsthesia and antisepsis, which were the joint foundation stones for the rapid advance of surgery. Neither of them would have been of much use without the other.

Nussbaum of Munich said in 1879:[18]

"Previous to 1875 the antiseptic system had not been tried, though carbolic and chlorine water had been freely used. Pyæmia struck down all compound fractures and nearly all amputations. . . . In 1872 hospital gangrene was

43

added to pyæmia. . . . Not one of his students had seen in the hospital an instance of union by first intention." . . . "In 1875, without any change in the wards, the nursing, the diet or the surroundings, Lister's antiseptic treatment was introduced. . . . " From that day there has not been one case of hospital gangrene, of pyæmia or of erysipelas."

Semmelweiss,[19] in Vienna, had reduced the mortality from puerperal fever in his clinic from 12 per cent. to 3 per cent. by insisting that his students wash their hands in chlorinated lime water. But no one would listen to this forerunner of Lister, and he died insane in 1865.

Many things which are usually thought to be later developments had their origin in the Victorian age. D. Lowson, assistant surgeon to the Hull Royal Infirmary, did a pneumonectomy in 1893,[20] many years before the rise of thoracic surgery. Corneal grafting was practised occasionally as early as 1879.[21] Tubeless tyres, which were introduced with a flourish of trumpets in the middle 1950s as something revolutionary, date from 1898.[22] Charles Lamont introduced a new process for drying eggs in 1868.[23] He claimed that 1,200 dehydrated eggs could be packed in the space of one cubic foot. This process only came into its own in the Battle of the Atlantic seventy years later.

Sir Thomas Watson suggested the use of rubber gloves in 1843,[24] to protect the surgeon rather than the patient, but rubber was then in its infancy and nothing further came of the idea. J. Williams, of Manchester,[25] was actually the first to use them. He said in Jan., 1871: "Some time ago, when in London, having to attend a woman who had been suffering from syphilis, I took the precaution of using an india-rubber glove, which Mr. Walters, of Moorgate Street, made for me." A few months later a country practitioner in Westmoreland, bearing the famous name of Liston,[26] was using them. After trying to make some himself two or three years before for use in confinements in syphilitic cases, he finally got some made in London.

Their introduction is usually attributed to W. S. Halsted, the American surgeon, about nineteen years later. One story is that he found that the skin of the hands could not be made sterile, another is that his theatre sister—whom he afterwards married—was allergic to the disinfectants used. In any case he was not the first to use them. John Ward Cousins, of Portsmouth, a man of many inventions, was using special operating coats in 1884.[27]

On the other hand some things thought to be long obsolete and extinct lingered on very late. As recently as 1872 seven United States soldiers were wounded by arrows in the Indian wars, five of them dying.

When the first X-ray picture was published in *The Lancet* on Jan. 25, 1896, a reference was made to that indefatigable inventor Sir Benjamin Ward Richardson, who had tried in 1868 to get a strong enough light to see through the human body, or parts of it. He used magnesium ribbon. Fortunately he lived long enough—until Nov., 1896—to hear the news that what he had tried to do was now possible.

In the 1890s the controversy about woman doctors was at its height. One sour critic commented that it was a horrible sight to see a woman operate. To which came the devastating reply from another correspondent that it was also a horrible sight to see some men operate!

The critics then said that women were incapable of arresting hæmorrhage by reason of their tendency to faint, to which the realistic reply was given that men often fainted in the medical schools, nurses rarely, if ever.

In 1907 there was an indignant letter from someone who suffered from excessive taxation—probably a man who remembered the 1870s when income tax was 2d. in the pound. "Sir,—The cruel and iniquitous income tax, which is apparently to be maintained at the war level of 1/-, weighs with special injustice on the medical man." To those of us who have long been accustomed to, if not enthusiastic about, an income tax of eight to nine times this amount, this letter only arouses a feeling of envy for somebody who didn't know when he was well off.

Two years later came another letter with a bitter complaint about the tax on petrol, which stood at the terrible figure of 3d. a gallon. We, who pay exactly ten times this amount on every gallon, merely have a feeling of mild astonishment that he bothered to waste a stamp on such a trivial matter.

In browsing through the old medical journals in search of items of anæsthetic interest one comes across instances of supreme courage and resolution. For example Mr. Lowson was bold and adventurous when he excised his first lung in 1893. The anæsthetic would almost certainly be chloroform on an open mask with no provision for endotracheal airways or for artificial inflation. Isaac Baker Brown was also a very resolute man who did not shrink from responsibility. He was born in 1812 in Essex, and qualified in 1834. After trying all known methods of treatment for ovarian cysts, including mercury, diuretics and tonics, tapping, tapping followed by pressure and iodine injections, he came to the conclusion that removal by ovariotomy was the only effective treatment. The risk was enormous, but the condition was eventually fatal by reason of its mere size, if it was treated in any other way. The early ovariotomists were contemptuously referred to as "belly rippers" by their less adventurous colleagues. His first three cases died—not an encouraging beginning. But he held fast to his opinion. He knew he was right —that the death rate did not matter in an inevitably fatal disease, but that any recoveries were lives saved. His fourth case, in 1852, was his own sister. She was still living, the mother of several children, when this man of iron died in 1873.

The steady advances of science and material prosperity during the nineteenth century led many Victorians to think that progress in all things was inevitable and automatic. We of the twentieth century are not so sure. It is true that science and social conditions have continued to progress with increasing acceleration and increasing complexity, but the nineteenth century never had anything like the horrors of Belsen and Auschwitz. And it had no problems comparable to the hydrogen bomb and the inter-continental ballistic missile.

Their scientists actually classified man as *Homo sapiens*—man the wise. How very foolish of them! Man the clever, if you like, man the brainy, man the intellectual, but not man the wise. Wisdom is very different from cleverness.

Any American citizen who feels superior or supercilious after reading about the appalling living conditions of English people in an age which was supposed to be progressive and prosperous would be well advised to consult the *Boston Medical and Surgical Journal*. It records a fatal case of puerperal sepsis in a negress who was sold at full term pregnancy just before Christmas—the time of peace and goodwill towards men.[28] "This woman was sold under a guarantee of soundness; under the circumstances, ought the buyer or the seller to be the loser?"

Wasn't there something about all men being created equal and that their unalienable rights included Life, Liberty and the pursuit of Happiness?[29]

REFERENCES

[1] *Lancet* (1908), Jan. 18. 191.

[2] *Lancet* (1846), Aug. 15. 172.

[3] *Lancet* (1846), Aug. 8. 166.

[4] *Lancet* (1860), Oct. 13. 365.

[5] *Lancet* (1900), Sept. 15. 856.

[6] *Med. Annu.* (1903). 951.

[7] *Lancet* (1908), Aug. 15. 495. Lionel F. West.

[8] *Lancet* (1846). I. 13.

[9] *Lancet* (1848), May 6. 488.

[10] *Lancet* (1922), Nov. 11. 1016.

[11] *Lancet* (1847). II. 185.

[12] C. T. Thackrah (1832). *The effects of arts, trades and professions . . . on health and longevity.* (233 pp.). 2nd Ed. London. Longman.

[13] *Lancet* (1883), Nov. 17. 868.

[14] *Lancet* (1888). Special Sanitary Commission on sweatshops. A series of articles.

[15] *Lancet* (1847), Aug. 21. 209.

[16] *Lancet* (1885), Aug. 15. 307.

[17] *Lancet* (1896), Jan. 18. 205.

[18] *Lancet* (1879), Oct. 18. 579.

[19] *Lancet* (1886), July 31, 206; and Aug. 7 246.

[20] *Brit. med. J.* (1893), June 3. 1152.

[21] *Med. Tms. Gaz.* (1879), Nov. 22. 579.

[22] *Med. Annu.* (1898) 627. Fleuss tubeless tyre for cycles.

[23] *Brit. med. J.* (1868), Jan. 4. 17.

[24] *Lancet* (1906), June 2. 1533.

[25] *Lancet* (1871), Jan. 14. 73.

[26] *Lancet* (1871), May 13. 673. Jas. Robt. Liston; Kirkby Stephen.

[27] *Brit. med. J.* (1884), April 19. 769.

[28] *Boston med. surg. J.* (1845), Sept. 3. Vol. 33. 99.

[29] United States' Declaration of Independence, July 4, 1776.

CHAPTER 3

THE BEGINNING OF THINGS

"To crib from one book is plagiarism, to crib from a dozen is research; to crib from any larger number will get you a doctorate of philosophy from one of the less exacting universities."

A. A. Thomson, *The Great Cricketer.*

THE first reference to anæsthesia in the medical press, so far as I know, occurs in the *Boston Medical and Surgical Journal,* on October 21st, 1846.[1]

"Strange stories are related in the papers of a wonderful preparation, in this city, by administering which, a patient is affected just long enough, and just powerfully enough, to undergo a surgical operation without pain."

A month later, in the same journal, there was something more definite than mere rumours.[2]

"In the leading article of this day's Journal, by Dr. H. J. Bigelow, the profession will notice that an impression exists here in Boston, that a remarkable discovery has been made. Unlike the farce and trickery of mesmerism, this is based on scientific principles, and is solely in the hands of gentlemen of high professional attainment, who make no secret of the matter or manner. To prevent it from being abused and falling into the power of low, evil-minded, irresponsible persons, we are informed that the discoverer has secured a patent, and that means were taken to have the same security in Europe even before publicity was given to it here. Without further remarks, we cheerfully publish all that has been given to us on the subject, and wait with impatience for the decision of the profession in regard to its real value."

All this, of course, was before the news of the great discovery had reached the Old World at all. The very first mention of anæsthesia on the European side of the Atlantic was a tiny paragraph in the weekly supplement to the *Liverpool Mercury* for Friday, December 18th, 1846.

"A method of mitigating pain in surgical operations by the inhalation of certain ethers has been discovered in America, and it is said that successful experiments have been made."

Dr. G. Chandler, Liverpool City Librarian, very kindly supplied me with this information when I was trying to track the movements of Dr. Fraser, one of the people who brought the news. The next reference,

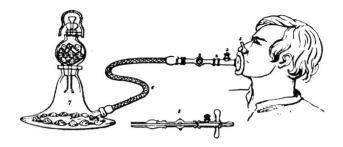

FIG. 12

Lancet, 1847, Jan. 2. 8. Also *Pharm. J., 1847, Jan. 353.* First use of ether in England. Francis Boott, Gower Street, London. "On Saturday, 19th Dec., 1846, a firmly fixed molar tooth was extracted in my study from Miss Lonsdale, by Mr. Robinson, in the presence of my wife, two of my daughters and myself, without the least sense of pain, or the movement of a muscle. . . ."

Five requisites are necessary to complete success and to avoid danger—viz.: First.—The air taken into the lungs should be exclusively that which has passed through the vessel of ether, and thus saturated with its vapour. Second.—The pad to be held over the mouth, to prevent any breathing of free atmosphere. Third.—The expired air to escape freely. Fourth.—The stopcock may be used to regulate the volume of the vapour of the ether at the commencement of the inhalation, and also to cut off the access of vapour to the mouth in cases of protracted operations, when it may be desirable to give the patient (in the state of insensibility) atmospheric air; and again to open the stopcock and let him breathe the vapour—thus lightening and deepening the degree of the sopor. Fifth.—The nasal spring is for compressing the nostrils during exhalation, and is to be taken off when the stopcock is closed for the breathing of atmospheric air, and again to be replaced when the vapour is inhaled.

The following explanation of the diagram will distinctly show, that in the construction of this apparatus these important requisites have been effected:

1. Pad for the mouth, which is held on by the operator or his attendant.
2. Horizontal valve for the escape of expired air, with a cap to be removed during inhalation.
3. Vertical flap valve.
4. Stopcock.
5. Nasal spring.
6. Elastic tube.
7. Glass vessels, stoppered and capped, containing small pieces of sponge saturated with ether.
8. Sectional view of the pad, showing the mouthpiece and pad.

A strong patient may require the larger glass stopper to be removed, but in ordinary cases the small stopper will be found sufficient.

The full effect of the vapour is generally produced in two or three minutes. Care should be taken that the mouthpiece during inhalation is perfectly horizontal, keeping the stopcock to the right hand, and the capped valve perpendicular.

49

and the first one in the medical press, is in *The Lancet*, under the date December 26th. On the very last page of the volume for the year 1846 is a single short and very non-committal paragraph:

"Dr. Bigelow, of Boston, U.S., has recently read a paper before one of the medical societies on a process for procuring insensibility to pain during surgical operations. Teeth in large numbers have been extracted, and even limbs amputated, without pain. Such a discovery, if it stands the test of examination, will be an invaluable boon. The means used is believed to be the inhalation of the vapour of sulphuric ether for two or three minutes, which it is stated, produces insensibility for about an equal length of time."

Exactly a week before this, on December 19th, Dr. Boott and Mr. Robinson had given ether for a dental extraction in Gower Street, London. This trial on Miss Lonsdale was a private trial of the method, and Mrs. Boott and her two daughters were the only spectators.

Two days afterwards, on December 21st, Liston amputated Frederick Churchill's leg under ether at University College Hospital. There was nothing private about this, but it was apparently too late to be written up in that week's issue. Liston's well-known operation is usually referred to as the first major operation under anæsthesia on this side of the Atlantic. But this is very doubtful.

There is one reference,[3] which is rarely mentioned in any of the books, which tends to show that it was not the first. For on the 19th December, the very same day as Dr. Boott and Mr. Robinson's pioneer dental anæsthesia, Dr. William Scott, surgeon to the Dumfries and Galloway Royal Infirmary, operated under ether on a patient in this hospital.

In a letter to the Editor of *The Lancet* Dr. William Scott says:

"Sir,—Dr. Vivian Poore, in his 'Clinical Remarks on chloroform and its administration,' published in your last number, states that Mr. Liston was the first person in this country to exhibit ether previous to an operation.

"I beg to state that I have a prior claim to Mr. Liston in this matter, as I exhibited ether on the 19th December, 1846, to a patient in the Dumfries and Galloway Royal Infirmary. My much esteemed and lamented friend, the late Sir J. Y. Simpson, having investigated the facts, with the statement I have made, was so satisfied with the authenticity of it that he not only in his lectures to the students attending his class, but also in his lecture on Anæsthetics delivered before the College of Surgeons in March, 1868, stated the priority of my claim to Mr. Liston.

"I may add that I received my information relative to the anæsthetic properties of ether from the late Dr. Fraser, surgeon of the Cunard steamer, which brought the important news from New York, and I operated as I have said within forty-eight hours of the discovery having been brought to this country. Your obedient servant, Wm. Scott, M.D., Surgeon to the Dumfries and Galloway Royal Infirmary, Dumfries, October 15th, 1872."

In the next week's issue is a reply from Dr. G. V. Poore.[4]

"Sir,—Dr. Wm. Scott, of Dumfries, in a letter on this subject in your last number, corrects me for stating, as he says 'that Mr. Liston was the first person in this country to exhibit ether previous to an operation'. If Dr. Scott refers again to my paper, he will find that my exact words were as follows: 'The first operation of magnitude which was performed under ether in this country was an amputation of the thigh by Liston'. A few lines before this he will see that I have given Mr. Robinson, the dentist, the credit of being the first in this country to employ ether as an anæsthetic. This was on the 19th December, the same day on which Dr. Scott exhibited ether. It would be interesting if Dr. Scott would tell us the nature of the operation to which his patient was subjected. I am, Sir, your obedient servant, G. V. Poore, Wimpole-street, October, 1872."

It would indeed be interesting, and I searched *The Lancet* for the next year or two with extra special care. But there was no reply from Dr. Scott. Perhaps he died soon after writing his first letter. In 1872 he would be at least 47—assuming that he was only 21 at the time of his first anæsthetic —and he may well have been very much older than this. At any rate there is no evidence available about the nature of the Dumfries operation. Nor could I find much more information about Dr. Scott or Dr. Fraser. On consulting a Scottish Medical Directory for 1845 at the National Library of Scotland in Edinburgh, I found that it was mainly composed of a list of names only. It was the first volume issued and was very incomplete. Addresses were hardly ever given and details of appointments were absent. So I could not identify with certainty any of the actors in this drama. All we can say with some certainty is that Dr. Scott and Mr. Robinson (with Dr. Boott) were the dead-heat pioneers in the use of ether, so far as Great Britain is concerned. Both of them used it two days before Liston.

Two points arise here for investigation. How did Dr. Scott get the news in this rather out of the way district, and secondly, how long did it take him, and the others, to put it into practice? Did they spend much time thinking it over and wondering whether it was safe to try it, or did they get down to the job quickly?

It must be remembered that there was no Atlantic cable at this date. That came later (August, 1858), so the news must have come by ship.

Dr. Scott is stated to have got the news forty-eight hours before his operation (that is on December 17th) from Dr. Fraser of the Cunarder which brought it across the ocean. Not knowing the duration of Atlantic voyages at that time, except that they were much longer than they are now, I wrote to the Cunard Company asking for information on this point. They replied:

"We thank you for your letter of August 7th (1958). We were very interested in the queries raised in your letter. We have established from our sailing records that the *Acadia*, one of the four wooden paddle steamers with which Samuel Cunard and his partners inaugurated their steamship services between Britain and North America in 1840, arrived at Liverpool on December 16, 1846. Her voyage took just under 14 days, the average approximate time taken by Atlantic steamers during the 1840's, the pioneer decade of the steamship on the North Atlantic. The date of the *Acadia's* arrival at Liverpool ties in with your theory that Dr. Fraser, the ship's surgeon, had passed on to Dr. Scott, of the Dumfries and Galloway Royal Infirmary, news of the first painless operations carried out in America.

"We have been unable to trace whether or not a Dr. Fraser was, in fact, the *Acadia's* surgeon at this time. Apart from captains, we have little record of the Company's early sea-going personnel.

"We hope this information will help you in your research work. If, from other sources, you are able to establish that the *Acadia's* ship's surgeon conveyed news of the first painless operations performed in America, we should, of course, very much like to have this interesting story confirmed."

A very helpful letter, as far as it goes. If the elusive Dr. Fraser could only be traced with certainty as an employee of the Company, their publicity department could make an interesting illustrated leaflet out of it!

I also wrote to several other sources enquiring about the duration of ocean crossings at that period. The information received was interesting, but of secondary importance only in view of the Cunard Company's definite statement about the *Acadia* and her voyage at the exact time in question. The Deputy Keeper of the South Kensington Science Museum stated:

". . . we have a note that in 1847 the Cunard P.S. (paddle steamer) *Hibernia* (1843), crossed from Halifax to Liverpool in 9 days 1 hour 30 minutes, at a mean speed of 11.67 knots. This was, however, a record at the time, for the normal service speed of the vessel is stated to have been about 9.25 knots."

A calculation from the time and average speed of this record crossing makes the distance of this particular voyage about 2,538 nautical miles,

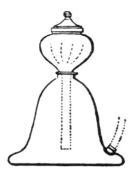

FIG. 13

Pharm. J., 1847, VI., Jan. 338. Apparatus for inhaling ether. This rough sketch of Squire's apparatus was published as soon as possible, before Squire's own description and picture of it.

"Mr. Squire has contrived an apparatus for this purpose. It resembles a Nooth's apparatus—a sponge wetted with ether being placed in the upper part, the vapour being heavier than atmospheric air, descends through the tube to the lower vessel, to which is attached a flexible tube and mouthpiece. In this tube there is a valve to prevent the expired air returning into the vessel. Mr. Squire informs us that the ether should be washed with water in order to purify it. The apparatus used in America was more simple, being more like an ordinary inhaler, with the valve in the tube near the mouthpiece. A common Mudge's inhaler, with the addition of the valve, would answer the purpose, in the absence of Mr. Squire's improved apparatus. The old plan of introducing a teaspoonful of ether into a bladder or silk bag, and inhaling it in the same manner as nitrous oxide gas, is not nearly so effectual as the above; since the same air is inhaled repeatedly, either with small additions, which dilute the ethereal vapour, or in a vitiated state, without the requisite oxygen. By means of the above apparatus, the supply of ethereal vapour mixed with a due proportion of fresh atmospheric air, is constant, and the effect is more uniform and speedy. We are informed that Dr. A. T. Thomson has been in the habit of exhibiting to his class the effects of ether when inhaled, in order to demonstrate the analogy in its effects with that of the nitrous oxide gas. The practice has recently been discontinued, as it was found to irritate the lungs of some persons, and in one case produced inflammation. Mr. Squire considers that this arose from the ether not having been previously washed with water."

if my arithmetic is correct. At her usual speed the *Hibernia* would therefore take about 11½ days over the trip. But time and speeds at that date were much more dependent on the weather than they are now. Engines were weak and not very trustworthy, and a good deal of reliance was still placed on the old and well-tried sails. One would imagine, too, that paddle wheels were highly vulnerable to Atlantic gales.

The Assistant Keeper of the National Maritime Museum at Greenwich stated:

"In answer to your letter, it appears that the winter of 1846 saw some very heavy storms in the Atlantic, and the *Great Western* for example took 24 days, 17th November to 12th December, to cross, in comparison with the normal fortnight or so."

So the chronology of events was something like this: 16th October—Morton's "ether day" demonstration, the anniversary of which is still celebrated at the Massachusetts General Hospital. 28th November—The date of Dr. Bigelow's letter to his friend, Dr. Boott. He apparently waited six weeks in order to make absolutely sure that the discovery was genuine before committing himself—a very commendable degree of restraint.

Allowing one day in the post in America, fourteen days for the voyage and one day for transmission of the letter to London, this gives a total of 59 days out of the 64 which elapsed from October 16th to December 19th. The remaining five days cannot be exactly accounted for. Perhaps the mails were slower than we have assumed.

If the letter, as is probable, arrived in the *Acadia* on the 16th December, it certainly could not have got to London before the 17th, which only left two days for Dr. Boott and Mr. Robinson to devise their inhaler and get it made by Mr. Hooper, and to procure supplies of ether, which of course was not readily available from stock at that time. Quite probably it had to be specially made. Or a few chemists might have had a small amount available, as it had occasionally been used as an inhalant in medical conditions.

The same timing applies to Dr. Scott in Dumfries. The *Acadia* arrived on December 16th, and Dr. Fraser (whether he was the ship's surgeon or a passenger is of no importance from this point of view) must have rushed home in a great hurry to give the news to Scott on the 17th or possibly the 18th. So very little time was lost in trying out the new discovery. The next task was to find out whether anything further could

54

be found out about the Scottish use of ether. The County Librarian of Dumfries-shire replied:

"We have on this occasion—and on previous occasions—searched the press for contemporary information on the first use of anæsthetics in Dumfries and Galloway Infirmary in 1846, but nothing appears to have been reported at the time. This is strange, because in 1846 and the early part of the following year the *Dumfries Courier* contained frequent references to the American discovery, one of which I enclose for your information.

"Extract from *Dumfries Courier*, January 11th, 1847:

"'An American discovery in surgery, rendering patients insensible by the respiration of Sulphuric Aether, so that operations might be performed without the accompaniment of pain, has attracted much attention in this country.

"'According to several statements which we have read, there is a strong probability of this proving successful, which will ensure its general adoption among the medical profession, who, whatever might have been the state of feeling at the time of the discovery of the circulation of the blood, are now eager enough to avail themselves of any improvement in their noble profession. Experiments have not been sufficiently made to satisfy all doubts on this subject; and particularly as to whether the respiration of the æther may not prove injurious to the permanent health of the patient. According to one account, it tends to put the patient in a sinking state, but this was counteracted by the application of wine'."

In the nineteenth century to sink was a common euphemism for dying. Many case reports ended wish the words "the patient sank," followed by an account of the post-mortem!

"The immense advantage of being able to perform the numerous severe operations necessary in surgery upon a patient in a state of unconsciousness are very obvious. The chief one is undoubtedly the avoidance of the dreadful pain endured by the hapless sufferer; and in many cases treatment may be resorted to, which was often withheld from the dread of inflicting suffering, doubtful in its results, or under which death, from the infliction, might have ensued. Moreover many skilful surgeons can never become good operators from the want of the great nerve required in this branch of their profession; but with the unconscious patient under his hands, the most sensitive medical man may apply the knife or the saw with ease and confidence."

The Librarian's letter continues:

"The story of Dr. Fraser bringing the news to Dumfries and of the operation carried out by Dr. Scott is, however, frequently quoted in later sources. I am sending herewith an extract from 'Local Parish Histories and new Statistical Account,' which appeared in the press of April 25th, 1876, in which you will

55

read an account of the incident. I am also sending on loan a copy of *The Dumfries and Galloway Royal Infirmary: a brief pictorial survey,* 1776-1948, which contains a further account. . . ."

Extract from *Local Parish Histories and New Statistical Account,* Dumfries, April 25th, 1876.

"It is remarkable that the first use of anæsthetics in an operation in Great Britain took place in the Dumfries Infirmary. The discovery was made in the United States. A Dr. Fraser, a native of the town, the surgeon of the Cunard steamer which brought the news to this country, came to Dumfries immediately after his ship arrived and gave the information of the discovery to his professional brethren there, who lost no time in making an experiment. On the 19th December, 1846, Dr. Scott, in the presence of Dr. McLachlan and his other colleagues, administered sulphuric ether to a patient in the Infirmary, and afterwards performed upon him a painless operation. The honour of being the first to use anæsthetics in this island has at various times been claimed by others, but it is now generally admitted that the Dumfries Infirmary was really the scene of its first use in this country."

The Secretary of the Dumfries and Galloway Hospital Board also replied very fully and courteously to my letter, and sent me another copy of the illustrated brochure on the history of the Royal Infirmary, Dumfries, from its foundation down to 1948, the date on which it ceased to be a voluntary hospital and was taken over by the National Health Service. He said:

"You information accords generally with that shown in a survey of the Infirmary published in 1948 as a valediction to the voluntary hospital, and a copy of which I enclose. You will note, I have no doubt, the suggestion that Dr. Scott operated at Dumfries somewhere about the end of October or the beginning of November, 1846, and some weeks before the similar use of the anæsthetic at University College Hospital, London. Unfortunately there is no case record of the Dumfries operation so far as I know, but its authenticity would not appear to be in doubt."

The booklet referred to by the Secretary claims the first administration of ether in Europe by a margin of several weeks.

"Towards the end of October or the beginning of November, 1846, Dr. Scott, assisted by Dr. McLauchlan, successfully carried out an amputation in a painless and satisfactory manner on a patient while he was in a complete state of insensibility as a result of the administration of sulphuric ether gas given by a Dr. Wm. Fraser (a surgeon in the Cunard Steamship Company and a son of James Fraser, a surgeon in Dumfries) then on a visit to his native town,

FIG. 14

Pharm. J., 1847, VI, Feb. 351.
Mr. Squire's own description and picture of his apparatus. A, The urn with its stopper, into which the ether is poured. B, Valve which admits the air. C, Contains sponge saturated with ether. D, Valve which opens at each inspiration, and closes at each expiration. E, Ferrule for regulating the quantity of atmospheric air admitted. G, Mouthpiece. H, Lower vase. I, Spring for closing the nose.

He suggested that all failures should be reported. In two cases of failure the nose was not held. He strongly advises washed ether.

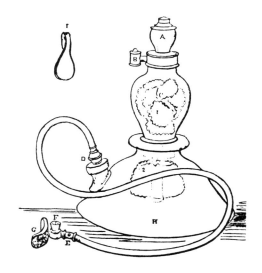

but whose sojourn in the United States had brought him into contact with Dr. W. T. G. Morton, of Boston, U.S.A.—sometimes hailed as the discoverer of anæsthesia—and from whom he learned of the effects of the inhalation of this gas. All that is known of the apparatus used is that it was an 'apparatus hastily improvised by Dr. Fraser,' and consequently there seems reason to believe that it would be similar to that used by Dr. Morton some weeks earlier in Boston. The next place in the Old World where a major operation was carried out under a similar anæsthetic was at University College Hospital, London, on December 21, 1846, about six weeks after the experiment in Dumfries. . . . "

While agreeing with the Secretary and the hospital brochure about the authenticity of the facts, I disagree with their dates, which do not correspond with those taken from other sources. October is impossibly early. Morton's demonstration did not take place until the 16th of that month. This date is absolutely certain. Add fourteen days for the news to cross the Atlantic, if it crossed immediately, long before Dr. Bigelow posted his letter and long before Dr. Fraser embarked in the *Acadia*, and the whole of October is accounted for. November is just physically possible, but there is no other evidence for it, and there is evidence against it. In view of the definite statements from other sources, the Dumfries Hospital brochure appears to claim rather too early a date. On the whole, Dr. Scott's dead-heat with Dr. Boott seems to be the most probable. After all, that is the date which Dr. Scott himself gives.

The next point to be considered is transport. Supposing Dr. Fraser arrived in Liverpool on the 16th December in the *Acadia*, was it physically possible for him to get to Dumfries before the 19th, with the transport facilities then available?

It was the time above all others when the railways were being built, in bits and pieces, all over the country, mostly by small companies which afterwards amalgamated. But at the beginning their ambitions did not extend beyond local needs. Several books on railway history were consulted, but they were very confusing. Little isolated railways were scattered over the map in all directions, with large and small gaps between them. One clear fact emerged from the chaos, that the railway from Liverpool certainly did not extend as far as Dumfries at the date in question. It was doubtful whether it reached as far north as Carlisle over the lofty and difficult Shap Fell summit.

The publicity officer of British Railways was appealed to on this point, and he stated that no railway existed between Liverpool and Dumfries at that time. It had been advanced from Lancaster to Oxenholme (near Kendal), and to Kendal itself by 22/9/1846, and from Oxenholme to Carlisle on 17/12/1846, which was the very day after the *Acadia* docked, to make matters more confused. Whether the line was open to public traffic on that day is not certain. Very often the opening day of any new stretch of railway line was a public ceremony, with a slow and solemn journey by top-hatted notables, finishing up with a not-so-solemn banquet with speeches and drinks.

So it is possible that Dr. Fraser could only get as far as Kendal by train, which would leave him about 75 miles to do by road. This would probably take him more than one day at that season of the year. Mail coaches took about four days to travel from York to London, which is about 196 miles. Still, if the ship docked early he could get to Kendal on the 16th and arrive home on the 18th December. Remember that then there were no stupid delays over passports and immigration officials. Those are purely modern futilities which did not then exist.

If he was lucky enough to gate-crash the first ceremonial train with his big news he could have got to Carlisle on the 17th, for the train left Liverpool Lime Street at 10.15 a.m. and arrived at Carlisle at 5.20 p.m. That would have left him only about thirty-two miles by road on the 18th. So the operation on the 19th was quite feasible in either case.

Another possible route was by sea. The publicity officer stated that there were steamer sailings from Trafalgar Dock, Liverpool, to Dumfries, the fares being 10/- and 5/-, according to class, which was reasonable enough. The distance between these two places by rail is 159 miles, and was probably more by sea. The only trouble was that the sailings only took place six times a month, or about every five days, so the chances were about four to one against Dr. Fraser being lucky enough to catch a boat immediately. There is no record of the time taken for the voyage, but one of the Railway history books states that sailings from Liverpool to Ardrossan, which is considerably further north, took 26½ hours,[5] so if Dr. Fraser was lucky he could have done the journey by sea in the time. What is certain is that he must have been bursting with the news and anxious to give his own town the very earliest opportunity of using the new method.

Although *The Lancet*, with its one non-committal paragraph, had missed a first-rate journalistic scoop in its last number for 1846, it had beaten the *Provincial Medical and Surgical Journal*, which was the precursor and ancestor of the *British Medical Journal*. This weekly did not mention the matter at all in 1846.

The Lancet recovered itself quickly, for with the first issue for 1847, dated January 2nd, the big news crashed out with a vengeance. First of all there was news straight from the horse's mouth. It started with a letter from Dr. Boott, enclosing Dr. Bigelow's letter from Boston, and a long paper by Bigelow, Junior, which summarised very carefully and efficiently all that was known about ether at that time.

Original Papers

Surgical Operations performed during insensibility produced by the inhalation of sulphuric ether.
Communicated by Francis Boott, M.D.

To the Editor of the *Lancet*,

Sir,—I beg to call your attention to the report of an anodyne process, by means of which surgical operations have been performed without pain. I think it would be interesting to the profession if published in the *Lancet*. I also send a letter from Dr. Bigelow, bearing date more than three weeks after the report drawn up by his son. I wish to add, that Dr. Bigelow is one of the first physicians of Boston, a Professor of the Medical School of Harvard College, and a man of great accomplishment.

Gower Street, Bedford Square.   Yours sincerely,

Dec., 1846.   F. Boott.

Extract from a private letter from Dr. Bigelow to Dr. Francis Boott:

Boston. Nov. 28, 1846.

My dear Boott,

        I send you an account of a new anodyne process lately introduced here, which promises to be one of the important discoveries of the present age. It has rendered many patients insensible to pain during surgical operations, and other causes of suffering. Limbs and breasts have been amputated, arteries tied, tumours extirpated, and many hundreds of teeth extracted, without any consciousness of the least pain on the part of the patient.

The inventor is Dr. Morton, a dentist of this city, and the process consists of the inhalation of the vapour of ether to the point of intoxication. I send you the *Boston Daily Advertiser*, which contains an article written by my son Henry, and which is extracted from a medical journal, relating to the discovery.

Let me give you an example. I took my daughter Mary, last week, to Dr. Morton's rooms, to have a tooth extracted. She inhaled the ether about one minute, and fell asleep instantly in the chair. A molar tooth was then extracted, without the slightest movement of a muscle or fibre. In another minute she awoke, smiled, said the tooth was not out, had felt no pain, nor had the slightest knowledge of the extraction. It was an entire illusion.

The newspaper will give you the details up to its date, since when other operations have been performed with uniform success.

Dr. F. Boott.

The following paper, by Henry Jacob Bigelow, M.D., one of the surgeons to the Massachusetts General Hospital, was read before the Boston Society of Medical Improvement, November 9th, 1846, an abstract having been previously read before the American Academy of Arts and Sciences, November 3rd, 1846:

It has long been an important problem in medical science, to devise some method of mitigating the pain of surgical operations. An efficient agent for this purpose has at length been discovered. A patient has been rendered completely insensible during an amputation of the thigh, regaining consciousness after a short interval. Other severe operations have been performed without the knowledge of the patients. So remarkable an occurrence will, it is believed, render the following details relating to the history and character of the process not uninteresting.

"Not uninteresting!" Surely the greatest masterpiece of understatement of all time, when one considers the shattering impact of this article on a world where pain was still, as it always had been, absolutely inseparable from surgery.

On the 16th of October, 1846, an operation was performed at the hospital, upon a patient who had inhaled a preparation administered by Dr. Morton, a dentist of this city, with the alleged intention of producing insensibility to pain. Dr. Morton was understood to have extracted teeth under similar circumstances, without the knowledge of the patient. The present operation was performed by Dr. Warren, and though comparatively slight, involved an incision near the lower jaw, of some inches in extent. During the operation the patient muttered, as in a semi-conscious state, and afterwards stated that the pain was considerable, though mitigated; in his own words, as though the skin had been scratched with a hoe. There was probably, in this instance, some defect in the process of inhalation, for, on the following day, the vapour was administered to another patient with complete success. A fatty tumour, of considerable size, was removed by Dr. Hayward from the arm of a woman, near the deltoid muscle. The operation lasted four or five minutes, during which time the patient betrayed occasional marks of uneasiness; but upon subsequently regaining her consciousness, professed not only to have felt no pain, but to have been insensible to surrounding objects—to have known nothing of the operation, being only uneasy about a child left at home. No doubt, I think, existed in the minds of those who saw this operation, that the unconsciousness was real; nor could the imagination be accused of any share in the production of these remarkable phenomena.

In this careful, factual, judicial account Henry Bigelow mentions failures, or partial failures, as they occur, but makes it clear that the procedure could be—and often was—most efficient, even in its experimental stage. Henry J. Bigelow was born on March 11th, 1818, qualified in 1841, and became surgeon to the hospital in 1846. He later became Professor of surgery at Harvard University. He died October 30th, 1890.

I subsequently undertook a number of experiments, with the view of ascertaining the nature of the new agent, and shall briefly state them, and also give some notice of the previous knowledge which existed of the use of the substances I employed.

The first experiment was with sulphuric ether, the odour of which was readily recognised in the preparation employed by Dr. Morton. Ether inhaled in vapour is well known to produce symptoms similar to those produced by the nitrous oxide. In my own former experience, the exhilaration has been quite as great, though perhaps less pleasurable, than that of this gas, or of the Egyptian *haschish* (extract of Indian hemp). It seemed probable that the ether might be so long inhaled as to produce excessive inebriation and insensibility; but in several experiments the exhilaration was so considerable that the subject became uncontrollable, and refused to inspire, through the apparatus. Experiments were next made with the oil of wine (ethereal oil). This is well known to be an ingredient in the preparation known as Hoffmann's anodyne, which also contains alcohol, and this was accordingly employed. Its effects upon the three or four subjects who tried it were singularly opposite to those of the ether alone. The patient was tranquillized and generally lost all inclination to speak or move. Sensation was partially paralyzed, though it was remarkable that consciousness was always clear, the patient desiring to be pricked or pinched, with a view to ascertain how far sensibility was lost. A much larger proportion of oil of wine, and also chloric ether, with and without alcohol, were tried, with no better effect.

It remains briefly to describe the process of inhalation by the new method, and to state some of its effects. A small, two-necked glass globe contains the prepared vapour, together with sponges, to enlarge the evaporating surface. One aperture admits the air to the interior of the globe, whence, charged with vapour, it is drawn through the second into the lungs. The inspired air thus passes through the bottle, but the expiration is diverted by a valve in the mouthpiece, and escaping into the apartment is thus prevented from vitiating the medicated vapour.

It is astonishing how many people designed ether inhalers with an uncomfortable and inefficient mouthpiece, as opposed to the far better facepiece. Even John Snow's first apparatus was designed in this way, though his second one about three months later was fitted with a proper facepiece, which he acknowledged to be an idea borrowed from Sibson. The idea of making the face-fitting a little larger, so as to include the nose, and of abolishing for ever the uncomfortable and inefficient nose-clip was such a little one, such an apparently obvious one, that it seems ridiculous that it was not used immediately, especially when one considers the amount of thought and ingenuity expended on many of these early models. The comfort of the patient appears to have been badly neglected here. Still, by the standards of the time, the patient was receiving such inestimable comfort and benefit from the prospect of painless surgery that little matters like an uncomfortable nose-clip tended to escape notice altogether. It is, after all, so easy to be wise after the event, so easy to pick last year's Derby winner! However, to continue with Henry Bigelow's report:

A few of the operations in dentistry, in which the preparation has as yet been chiefly applied, have come under my observation. The remarks of the patients will convey an idea of their sensations.

A boy of sixteen, of medium stature and strength, was seated in the chair. The first few inhalations occasioned a quick cough, which afterwards subsided; at the end of eight minutes the head fell back, and the arms dropped, but owing to some resistance in opening the mouth, the tooth could not be reached before he awoke. He again inhaled for two minutes, and slept for three minutes, during which time the tooth, an inferior molar, was extracted. At the moment of extraction the features assumed an expression of pain, and the hand was raised. Upon coming to himself he said he had had a "first rate dream—very quiet," he said, "and had dreamed of Napoleon—had not the slightest consciousness of pain—the time had seemed long"; and he left the chair, feeling no uneasiness of any kind, and evidently in a high state of admiration. The pupils were dilated during the state of unconsciousness, and the pulse rose from 130 to 142.

Evidently no prop or gag was used in this case. One or two gags were designed in the pre-anæsthetic era for operations far back in the mouth, but dentists were not in the habit of using them in conscious patients, any more than dentists do today with local anæsthesia. The patient was expected to keep his own mouth open. The first dental prop designed for anæsthesia was that of F. B. Imlach in 1847.

Mr. J. Chitty Clendon, in a pamphlet *On the use of chloroform in dental surgery,* published in 1849, pointed out its disadvantages in ordinary dental cases. The patient slips down in the chair, there is jaw-clenching, and gags are not satisfactory as they alarm the patient and generally slip out of position. Respiration is also more difficult with the mouth propped open. Also there is difficulty in estimating the length of the operation and in deciding how much chloroform to give. He evidently does not contemplate any method of continuous administration.

Mr. Clendon admits that chloroform is useful in difficult cases, but is not enthusiastic about it for routine use. This is his considered opinion, and not mere prejudice, because he was one of the very earliest in the field when ether was first used. He described his own inhaler three weeks after Dr. Boott's first case. So he was willing enough to try new ideas, but honest enough to point out their disadvantages and dangers, which, in his department, took many years to overcome.

A girl of sixteen immediately occupied the chair. After coughing a little, she inhaled during three minutes, and fell asleep, when a molar tooth was extracted, after which she continued to slumber tranquilly during three minutes more. At the moment when force was applied, she flinched and frowned, raising her hand to her mouth, but she said she had been dreaming a pleasant dream, and knew nothing of the operation.

A stout boy of twelve, at the first inspiration coughed considerably, and required a good deal of encouragement to induce him to go on. At the end of three minutes from the first fair inhalation, the muscles were relaxed, and the pupil dilated. During the attempt to force open the mouth he recovered his consciousness, and again inhaled during two minutes, and in the ensuing one minute two teeth were extracted, the patient seeming somewhat conscious, but upon actually awaking he declared "it was the best fun he ever saw," avowed his intention to come there again, and insisted upon having another tooth extracted upon the spot. A splinter which had been left afforded an opportunity of complying with his wish, but the pain proved to be considerable. Pulse at first 110, during sleep 96, afterwards 144; pupils dilated.

This patient is stated to have been relaxed at the end of three minutes—with no pre-medication. Hardly, I think. That he was not relaxed is made clear in the next sentence, for the jaw was so resistant that the tooth could not be extracted.

The next patient was a healthy-looking, middle-aged woman, who inhaled the vapour for four minutes; in the course of the next two minutes a back molar tooth was extracted, and the patient continued smiling in her sleep for three minutes more. Pulse 120, not affected at the moment of the operation, but smaller during sleep. Upon coming to herself, she exclaimed that "it was beautiful—she dreamed of being at home—it seemed as if she had been gone a month."

These cases, which occurred successively in about an hour, at the rooms of Dr. Morton, are fair samples of the average results produced by the inhalation of the vapour, and will convey an idea of the feelings and expressions of many of the patients subjected to the process. Dr. Morton states, that in upwards of two hundred patients, similar effects have been produced. The inhalation, after the first irritation has subsided, is easy, and produces a complete unconsciousness at the expiration of a period varying from two to five or six, sometimes eight minutes; its duration varying from two to five minutes; during which the patient is completely insensible to the ordinary tests of pain. The pupils in the cases I have observed have been generally dilated; but with allowance for excitement and other disturbing influences, the pulse is not affected, at least in frequency; the patient remains in a calm and tranquil slumber, and wakes with a pleasurable feeling. The manifestation of consciousness or resistance I at first attributed to the reflex function, but I have since had cause to modify this view.

It is natural to inquire whether no accidents have attended the employment of a method so wide in its application and so striking in its results. I have been unable to learn that any serious consequences have ensued. One or two robust patients have failed to be affected. I may mention as an early and unsuccessful case, its administration in an operation performed by Dr. Hayward, where an elderly woman was made to inhale the vapour for at least half an hour without effect. Though I was unable at the time to detect any imperfection in the process, I am inclined to believe that such existed. One woman became much excited, and required to be confined to the chair. As this occurred to the same patient twice, and in no other case as far as I have been able to learn, it was evidently owing to a peculiar susceptibility.

By this time Morton had done over 200 cases, which was just about the total world-experience of anæsthesia at that time. Accidents, in the sense of fatalities, there were none. Barring very bad luck they were hardly to be expected in this small number of cases dealt with by an inherently safe drug like ether. There was never any question of over-dosage—in fact, hardly any of these patients ever reached the stage of surgical anæsthesia, as we know it. A few failures are described, due to lack of pre-medication, crude apparatus and lack of experience, all factors which weighed the balance very heavily in favour of light anæsthesia. Any tough or resistant patient was almost necessarily a failure under these conditions. The next case to be described is probably the only one in the whole series who was ever properly under!

Very young subjects are affected with nausea and vomiting, and for this reason Dr. Morton has refused to administer it to children. Finally, in a few cases, the patient has continued to sleep tranquilly for eight or ten minutes, and once, after a protracted inhalation, for the period of an hour.

The following case, which occurred a few days since, will illustrate the probable character of future accidents. A young man was made to inhale the vapour, while an operation of limited extent, but somewhat protracted duration, was performed by Dr. Dix upon the tissues near the eye. After a good deal of coughing, the patient succeeded in inhaling the vapour, and fell asleep at the end of about ten minutes. During the succeeding two minutes, the first incision was made, and the patient awoke, but unconscious of pain. Desiring to be again inebriated, the tube was placed in his mouth and retained there about twenty-five minutes, the patient being apparently half affected, but as he subsequently stated, unconscious. Respiration was performed partly through the tube, and partly with the mouth open. Thirty-five minutes had now elapsed, when I found the pulse suddenly diminishing in force, so much so, that I suggested the propriety of desisting. The pulse continued decreasing in force, and from 120 had fallen to 96. The respiration was very slow, the hands cold and the patient insensible. Attention was now, of course, directed to the return of respiration and circulation. Cold affusions, as directed for poisoning with alcohol, were applied to the head, the ears were syringed, and ammonia presented to the nostrils and administered internally. For fifteen minutes the symptoms remained stationary, when it was proposed to use active exercise, as in a case of narcotism from opium. Being lifted to his feet, the patient soon made an effort to move his limbs, and the pulse became more full, but again decreased in the sitting posture, and it was only after being compelled to walk during half an hour that the patient was able to lift his head. Complete consciousness returned only at the expiration of an hour. In this case the blood was flowing from the head, and rendered additional loss of blood unnecessary;

indeed the probable hæmorrhage was previously relied on as salutary in its tendency.

This is the first case on record in which resuscitation methods were considered necessary. As far as one can judge from the description there was really no cause for alarm. This anæsthetic was much longer than the ordinary two or three minute analgesia which was usual at that time, and the patient naturally took longer to recover.

Two recent cases serve to confirm, and one, I think, to decide, the great utility of this process: on Saturday, November 7th, at the Massachusetts General Hospital, the right leg of a young girl was amputated above the knee, by Dr. Hayward, for disease of the joint. Being made to inhale the preparation, after protesting her inability to do so, from the pungency of the vapour, she became insensible in about five minutes. The last circumstance she was able to recall was the adjustment of the mouthpiece of the apparatus, after which she was unconscious until she heard some remark at the time of securing the vessels—one of the last steps of the operation. Of the incision she knew nothing, and was unable to say, upon my asking her, whether or not the limb had been removed. She refused to answer several questions during the operation, and was evidently completely insensible to pain or other external influences. This operation was followed by another, consisting of the removal of a part of the lower jaw, by Dr. Warren. The patient was insensible to the pain of the first incision, though she recovered her consciousness in the course of a few minutes.

The character of the lethargic state which follows this inhalation is peculiar. The patient loses his individuality, and awakes after a certain period, either entirely unconscious of what has taken place, or retaining only a faint recollection of it. Severe pain is sometimes remembered as being of a dull character, sometimes the operation is supposed to be performed by somebody else. Certain patients whose teeth have been extracted, remember the application of the extracting instruments; yet none have been conscious of any real pain.

As before remarked, the phenomena of the lethargic state are not such as to lead the observer to infer this insensibility. Almost all patients under the dentist's hands scowl or frown; some raise the hand. The patient whose leg was amputated, uttered a cry when the sciatic nerve was divided. Many patients open the mouth, or raise themselves in the chair, upon being directed to do so. Others manifest the activity of certain intellectual faculties. An Irishman objected to the pain that he had been promised an exemption from it.

A young man taking his seat in the chair and inhaling a short time, rejected the globe, and taking from his pockets a pencil and card, wrote and added figures. Dr. Morton supposing him to be affected, asked if he would now submit to the operation, to which the young man willingly assented. A tooth was accordingly extracted, and the patient soon after recovered his senses. In none of these cases had the patients any knowledge of what had been done during their sleep.

I am, as yet, unable to generalise certain other symptoms to which I have directed attention. The pulse has been, as far as my observation extends, unaltered in frequency, though somewhat diminished in volume, but the excitement preceding an operation has, in almost every instance, so accelerated the pulse that it has continued rapid for a length of time. The pupils are, in a majority of cases, dilated; yet they are in certain cases unaltered, as in the above case of amputation.

The idea that the size of the pupils might vary with the depth of anæsthesia had not yet dawned. In fact the very idea of deep anæsthesia itself was not yet born.

The duration of the insensibility is another important element in the process. When the apparatus is withdrawn, at the moment of unconsciousness, it continues, upon the average, two or three minutes, and the patient then recovers completely or incompletely, without subsequent ill-effects. In this sudden cessation of the symptoms, this vapour in the air tubes differs in its effects from the narcotics or stimulants in the stomach, and as far as the evidence of a few experiments of Dr. Morton goes, from the ethereal solution of opium when breathed. Lassitude, headache and other symptoms, lasted for several hours when this agent was employed.

But if the respiration of the vapour be prolonged much beyond the first period, the symptoms are more permanent in their character. In one of the first cases, that of a young boy, the inhalation was continued during the greater part of ten minutes, and the subsequent narcotism and drowsiness lasted more than an hour. In a case alluded to before, the narcotism was complete during more than twenty minutes; the insensibility approached to coma.

The process is obviously adapted to operations which are brief in their duration, whatever be their severity. Of these, the two most striking are, perhaps, amputations and the extraction of teeth. In protracted dissections, the pain of the first incision alone is of sufficient importance to induce its use; and it may hereafter prove safe to administer it for a length of time, and to produce a narcotism of an hour's duration. It is not unlikely to be applicable in cases requiring a suspension of muscular action, such as the reduction of dislocations or of strangulated hernia; and finally, it may be employed in the alleviation of functional pain, of muscular spasm, as in cramp and colic, and as a sedative and narcotic.

This forecast of its use to obtain muscular relaxation is a remarkable feat of imagination. Nothing that Bigelow had seen could have suggested it to him. For none of these early cases ever reached the third stage of anæsthesia, much less its deeper planes.

The application of the process to the performance of surgical operations is, it will be conceded, new. If it can be shown to have been occasionally resorted to before, it was only an igorance of its universal application, and immense practical utility, that prevented such isolated facts from becoming generalised.

This must be a reference to Horace Wells' inconclusive demonstration at the hospital two years before. Crawford W. Long and other aspirants for priority had not yet put forward their claims. It might also be a belated acknowledgment that Wells had in fact used his gas successfully in some cases, even though his demonstration was abortive.

It is natural to inquire with whom this invention originated. Without entering into details, I learn that the patent bears the name of Dr. Charles T. Jackson, a distinguished chemist, and of Dr. Morton, a skilful dentist, of this city, as inventors—and has been issued to the latter gentleman as proprietor.

It has been considered desirable by the interested parties that the character of the agent employed by them should not be at this time announced; but it may be stated that it has been made known to those gentlemen who have had occasion to avail themselves of it.

I will add, in conclusion, a few remarks upon the actual position of this invention as regards the public.

No one will deny that he who benefits the world should receive from it an equivalent. The only question is, of what nature shall the equivalent be? Shall it be voluntarily conceded by the world, or levied upon it? For various reasons, discoveries in high science have been usually rewarded indirectly by fame, honours, position, and occasionally, in other countries, by funds appropriated for the purpose. Discoveries in medical science, whose domain approaches so nearly that of philanthropy, have been generally ranked with them; and many will assent with reluctance to the propriety of restricting by letters patent the use of an agent capable of mitigating human suffering. There are various reasons, however, which apologise for the arrangement, which I understand to have been made with regard to the application of the new agent.

1st. It is capable of abuse, and can readily be applied to nefarious ends.

2nd. Its action is not yet thoroughly understood, and its use should be restricted to responsible persons.

3rd. One of its greatest fields is the mechanical art of dentistry, many of whose processes are by convention, secret, or protected by patent rights. It is specially with reference to this art that the patent has been secured. We understand, already, that the proprietor has ceded its use to the Massachusetts General Hospital, and that his intentions are extremely liberal with regard to the medical profession generally; and that as soon as necessary arrangements can be made for publicity of the process, great facilities will be offered to those who are disposed to avail themselves of what now promises to be one of the important discoveries of the age.

But Bigelow's article was by no means all. Good though it was, it was hearsay, imported evidence only. But the amazing news continued to gather momentum in this, the most eventful number of *The Lancet* ever published. For there was a second letter from Dr. Boott, which not only quoted the opinion of the President of Harvard, but reported his own (and Mr. Robinson's) first case. Furthermore, Dr. Boott enclosed a letter from the great Robert Liston briefly recounting his first two cases. And on the same page there was a letter from Mr. Dorr, the agent for Morton's patent. All these are interesting enough to quote in full.

To the Editor of *The Lancet*—

Sir,—I forwarded a few days ago, for publication in *The Lancet*, Dr. H. J. Bigelow's report on the anodyne effects of the inhalation of the vapour of strong, pure sulphuric ether; and since that time I have received an address, delivered by the Hon. Edward Everett (late Minister from the United States to the court of St. James's), at the opening of the new Medical College in Boston, an extract from which will be interesting, as affording his high testimony to the safety and efficiency of the process. In a note, Mr. Everett, the President of Harvard College, says—"I am not sure that, since these remarks were delivered, a discovery has not been announced which fully realises the predictions of the text. I allude to the discovery of a method of producing a state of temporary insensibility to pain, by the inhalation of a prepared vapour. I witnessed a very successful instance of its application, on the 18th of November, and was informed at that time by Dr. Morton, that he had employed it in several hundred cases of dentistry. It has also been made use of with entire success at the Massachusetts General Hospital, and elsewhere in Boston, in capital operations of surgery. The few cases of failure may, perhaps, be ascribed to irregularities in the process of inhalation, or to peculiarities of temperament or constitution on the part of the patient. I understand that great confidence is placed in the discovery by the most distinguished members of the medical profession of this vicinity, and that they are disposed to regard it as an effectual method of inducing complete insensibility, under the most cruel operations, by means easily applied, entirely controllable, and productive of no subsequent bad consequences. It seems not easy to overrate the importance of such a discovery."

Mr. Everett was prolix and verbose, and took a long time to say very little. Was it not he who spoke for two hours at the dedication of the battlefield of Gettysburg seventeen years later? His introductory oration on that occasion was followed by that of the President of the United States, a gawky, ungainly, self-educated solicitor from the backwoods of Illinois. Abraham Lincoln spoke with the tongues of men and of angels —for two minutes—and one of the two speakers became immortal.

But Dr. Boott has not yet finished. The best part of his letter is yet to come—his personal experience.

I beg to add that on Saturday, the 19th, a firmly fixed molar tooth was extracted in my study from Miss Lonsdale, by Mr. Robinson, in the presence of my wife, two of my daughters and myself, without the least sense of pain, or the movement of a muscle. The whole process of inhalation, extracting and waking, was over in three minutes, yet the same apparatus was used in three or four cases afterwards, and failed in each case to produce insensibility. I attribute the failure to the defect in the valve of the mouthpiece, by which the expired air was returned to the bottle, instead of passing into the room. The valve was a ball and socket one, and required a very strong expiration to make it act freely. I would add that the efficiency of any apparatus must depend on the facility of breathing the vapour, and the perfect action of the valve. admitting the expired air to pass easily into the room. In Miss Lonsdale's case, we all observed she breathed strongly, and thus, no doubt, opened the valve. In all the other cases, we had great difficulty in making the patients breathe through the mouthpiece.

Gower Street.   Yours sincerely,

Dec. 21, 1846.   F. Boott.

Gower Street.

To the Editor of *The Lancet*.   Dec. 22nd, 1846.

Sir,—If you have not heard of Mr. Liston's success in the use of the inhaled ether, the following note I have received from him will interest you, as confirming the American report.

Clifford Street,

Dec. 21, 1846.

My dear Sir,—I tried the ether inhalation to-day in a case of amputation of the thigh, and in another requiring evulsion of both sides of the great toe nail, one of the most painful operations in surgery, and with the most perfect and satisfactory results.

It is a very great matter to be able thus to destroy sensibility to such an extent, and without, apparently, any bad result. It is a fine thing for operating surgeons, and I thank you most sincerely for the early information you were so kind as to give me of it.

Yours faithfully,

To Dr. Boott.   Robert Liston.

I hope Mr. Liston will report of these cases more fully.

Yours sincerely, F. Boott.

Liston might have added, one would think, that it was also a fine thing for the patient!

To the Editor of *The Lancet:*

Sir,—Having noticed, in several periodicals and newspapers, reports of two operations recently performed by Mr. Liston, at the University College Hospital, upon patients under the anodyne influence of inhaled vapour of ether, in which amputation of the thigh in one case, and evulsion of the nail of the great toe in the other case, were effected, without pain to the patients, I take the earliest opportunity of giving notice, through the medium of your columns, to the medical profession, and to the public in general, that the process for procuring insensibility to pain by the administration of the vapour of ether to the lungs, employed by Mr. Liston, is patented for England and the Colonies, and that no person can use that process, or any similar one, without infringing upon rights legally secured to others.

I am aware that doubts exist in the minds of some as to the liberality of rendering inventions or improvements, which tend to alleviate suffering, subjects of patents; but I cannot see why the individual who, by skill and industry, invents or discovers the means of diminishing, or, as in this instance, annihilating, human suffering, is not full as much entitled to compensation as he who makes an improvement in the manufacture of woollen or other fabrics. Indeed he is entitled to greater compensation, and for a stronger reason—he has conferred upon mankind a greater benefit.

With this view, I have accepted from the American inventors, or their representatives, the agency of affairs connected with the English patent; and it is my intention, while I hold the trust, to adhere to such a course, that the charge of illiberality shall rest upon any persons rather than upon the proprietors of the patent, or upon their agent.

James A. Dorr.

Dec. 28, 1846.   Duke Street, St. James's.

These, then, were the bombs which exploded into the placid world of 1847, on the second day of the year. Quite unheralded, except for the short paragraph on the last page of the 1846 volume. It marked the boundary between crude, brutal, stone-age surgery which had practically made no progress at all in the whole of recorded history, and a rapidly expanding and increasingly successful science.

The immediate effect was not so good as it appeared to be at first, not so good in practice as it was in theory. For, with a promise of painless surgery, surgeons became more ready to operate and patients more ready to submit to operations. This was a very risky business at that time. There was, of course, no major surgery as we know it—for the abdomen and thorax were forbidden ground, but the overall mortality of the minor surgery then practised ranged from ten to twenty per cent., or even more. The number of operations increased enormously and with this increase came a much larger number of deaths. Not for another twenty years was surgery really ready to expand. Not until Lister, the greatest of all Scottish surgeons—he was an Englishman, by the way—did it begin to get less hazardous. For until 1867 it remained, though less painful, the dirty, dangerous surgery of old, when infection was the normal occurrence after any wound. Brilliant technicians like Liston or Syme could be very dangerous men.

In the pre-anæsthetic era the number of operations in the large hospitals was about fifty a year. Not one of the London hospitals had more than one operating session a week. In 1825 *The Lancet* said of St. Thomas's Hospital—"The only operation performed here this week was that of lithotomy, by Mr. Tyrrell. . . . The operation was completed in about three minutes."

By 1862, after anæsthesia was well established, but before the coming of clean surgery, the numbers rose to about seven per week. St. Bartholomew's, in this year, had 329 operations with 32 deaths. Guy's had 541 with 44 deaths. Leeds General Infirmary had 211 operations with 16 deaths in 1861, none of them, of course, abdominals. By 1868, at the very beginning of Listerism, St. Bartholomew's actually had two operating sessions per week, and 534 operations with 60 deaths.

In the Index to Volume I for the first six months of 1847 there are no less than one hundred and eleven references to ether. Never before or since has such interest in anything been aroused. The issue for January 9th began quietly with a clinical lecture on dysentery, continued with a report of a case of simple and phlegmonous erysipelas, an account of a new pharmaceutical preparation, the syrup of iodide and chloride of iron, and then launched into a blistering leading article about an Edinburgh professor who was suspected of lapsing into the heresy of homoeopathy. Then came the first repercussions of Dr. Bigelow's news.

The indefatigable Dr. Boott weighs in with another letter, referring to Mr. Dorr's warning about patent infringements. He had taken the trouble and incurred the expense of getting Counsel's opinion, and getting it quickly:

" . . . as notice has been given of a patent for the inhalation of ether in surgical operations, and as such notice may deter surgeons and dentists from using it in the mitigation of pain, I beg to ask your insertion of the following letter, which I have received from one of Her Majesty's council (sic) 'learned in the law'.

" 'I am clearly of the opinion no patent can be valid, giving the patentee the exclusive privilege of administering the vapour of ether to the lungs. . . . I am satisfied you may safely advise your professional friends to continue the use of ether in their operations, without the slightest fear of legal consequences.'"

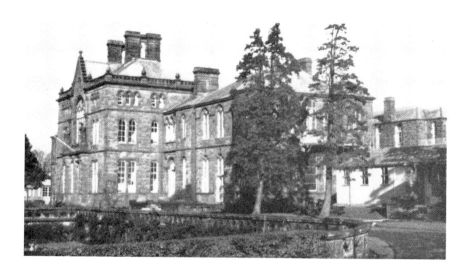

PLATE XII

Dumfries and Galloway Royal Infirmary, Dumfries. Photograph taken by the author, 1958. Here Dr. William Scott used ether on the same day as Dr. Boott and Mr. Robinson in London, on 19th Dec., 1846; two days before Liston used it in what is usually stated to be the first surgical operation under ether in the country.

FIG. 15

Lancet, 1847, Jan. 9. 50. Also *Pharm. J., 1847, VI. Feb. 354.* Mr. J. Chitty Clendon. Lecturer on Dental Surgery, Westminster Hospital. Ether apparatus, made by Mr. Clarke, philosophical instrument maker, Strand. Nine dental cases were reported, done with this model. Four of them were successful, four failures and one doubtful. Note the very small diameter and long length of the breathing tubes. There would be great frictional resistance. Note also the very small vapourising surface. It is surprising that there were any successes at all.

A, Ether and air tube; B, Inhaling tube with stopcock and valves. C, Mouthpiece; D, Ether, E, Glass cylinder, with brass fittings at the top.

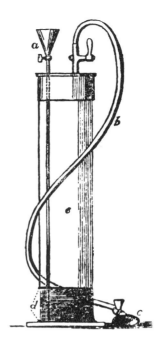

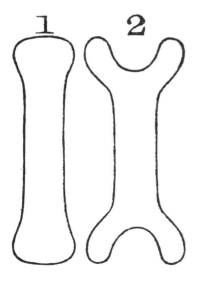

FIG. 16

Lancet, 1847, Dec. 18. 662. F. B. Imlach's dental prop. Made of ivory in different sizes. 1, Front view; 2, Side view.

Francis Brodie Imlach, F.R.C.S.Ed., born 1829. Qualified 1841. One time President of the Royal College of Surgeons of Edinburgh. Practised as a dentist. Died suddenly in the street on Christmas Eve, 1892.

The prop was placed between the bicuspids, or between the incisors if teeth had to be extracted from both sides. It was designed for chloroform, to avoid the difficulty that all dentists then complained of in getting the mouth open quickly during insensibility. "Ten to twelve inspirations are usually enough." No wonder there was frequent difficulty.

Counsel added that instruments and apparatuses for giving the ether might be patentable.

Mr. J. Chitty Clendon, Lecturer on Dental Surgery at the Westminster Hospital, describes nine dental cases under ether, apparently with 33% of successful results. On looking at the picture of the apparatus he used, one designed by himself, one marvels that the results even reached this standard. The small evaporating surface of the ether and the very narrow calibre of the breathing tubes were grave defects.

Next comes a claim for priority in the use of ether inhalation from Robert H. Collyer, M.D., of St. Helier, Jersey, who stated that he had not only tried it but published his results as far back as 1843. He did not claim to have used it for surgery, but stated that he had produced unconsciousness with it.

The following issue (January 16th) is even more occupied with the new discovery, almost monopolised by it, in fact. Mr. Squire described his apparatus to the Pharmaceutical Society, followed by Mr. Hooper, who constructed the apparatus used by Dr. Boott. There was a leading article of 3½ columns about ether, followed by a picture of Mr. Hooper's inhaler. Next came five columns of descriptions of operations, under the incredible and unprecedented heading, "Operations without Pain." Twenty-seven cases were recorded, from King's College Hospital, Guy's, the Westminster, St. Thomas's, Bristol General Hospital, Wolverhampton and the Western Institution for Diseases of the Eyes. Mr. J. Chitty Clendon writes again, and there is a further letter from Mr. Dorr, the patent agent, replying to Counsel's opinion.

No counsel can give a client valuable or even safe advice as to the validity of a patent, and danger of infringement, who has not read the specification, and does not know the claim of the patent. The patent for the Letheon has been duly sealed; but the specification is not yet made public.

Then there was an account of a meeting of the Westminster Medical Society, almost entirely devoted to reports of operations under ether and to Dr. Snow's researches into ether vapourisation. Thus early did John Snow jump on the bandwaggon.

Finally a small paragraph records the veterinary use of ether in Liverpool for an operation on a dog. The veterinarians were by no means backward in the field of anæsthesia, as can be seen from some of the early pictures. Mr. Hooper marketed a horse inhaler in September, 1847.

A week later, on January 23rd, Mr. J. B. Kington, Barrister, writes that:

" . . . a patent degrades a noble discovery to the level of a quack medicine. No extent of legal ingenuity could frame a specification which could prevent a medical man from procuring insensibility by administering ether, or from . . . performing any . . . surgical operation during such insensibility. . . . You cannot have a patent of a principle. . . . Can you patent the administration of jalap till a given effect is produced on the bowels? . . . If indeed the dicoverer has any novel method of generating the gas, or any novel apparatus for administering it, both may be patented. . . . "

Nothing more was heard about the patent, in this country at any rate.

An illustration of Snow's first warm ether apparatus appeared in this issue, designed, constructed, drawn and made into a woodcut in a very short space of time. Snow was well prepared for the new invention; he had been interested in the physiology of respiration for some years, and had published three long articles on the subject. Others looked upon anæsthesia solely as a means to an end—which, of course, it is. But it is fair to say that Snow was the only man to see it as a subject worthy of study in its own right. And this also was—and still is—true. And so it aroused his immediate interest, which lasted for the rest of his life.

There was at first great confusion and uncertainty about the name to be given to the new process. Not until Oliver Wendell Holmes, at Morton's request, created the new word anæsthesia and its adjective anæsthetic did anyone know what to call it. The exact date of birth of these words is uncertain, but it was very early, for Simpson used them when he announced his discovery of the effects of chloroform on 10th November, 1847.

Before this a great many synonyms were used, some of them clumsy and some of them cacophonous:

narcotism	hebetization
anæsthism	somniferous agent
stupefaction	soporized state
etherial state	apathisation
sopor	æthereal inhalation
etherization	etherification
anodyne process	lethargic state
ætherialisation	ætherization
soporization	æthereal influence
letheonization	anæstheticization

All these words were used, and a little later

chloroformism	chloroformised
chloroformization	chloroformal insensibility

The need for a new term was emphasised to the point of absurdity when the word etherization was used with reference to cases which were, by the context, conducted with the aid of chloroform alone.

Since writing the above I have discovered that Oliver Wendell Holmes did not actually create the word anæsthesia, because it already existed. It was used over a year before Morton's demonstration, in describing a case of partial anæsthesia of the legs, due to some medical condition, and of course nothing to do with inhalation anæsthesia.[6]

Holmes himself appears to have thought that he invented the word *de novo*. In 1886 he said to Edgar Willett:[7]

"Do you know the origin of the term (anæsthesia)?"
"No."
"I will tell you. I believe it was I who invented it, and this is how it occurred. Many years ago, when ether and chloroform were only just coming into use, Morton, the dentist of Boston, who was largely responsible for the introduction of ether, came to me and asked me if I could suggest for him a word which would describe the effect produced by their inhalation. After trying two or three words, æsthetic occurred to me as meaning sensitive, and in consequence anæsthetic as being insensitive easily followed, with anæsthesia for the condition produced. That," he concluded, "was, I believe, the origin of the term."

In *The Lancet* for the second half of 1847, the number of references to ether drops from 111 to 24. There are also 14 references to chloroform after the publication of Simpson's article on November 20th. In 1848 there is a drastic reversal of interest. Ether falls to 4 references, as opposed to 121 about its new rival. The early flood of ether inhalers ceased suddenly and was replaced by a steady output of chloroform masks and drop bottles.

REFERENCES

[1] *Boston med. surg. J.* (1846), Oct. 21. Vol. 35. 247.

[2] *Ibid.* Nov. 18. Vol. 35 324.

[3] *Lancet* (1872), Oct. 19. 585.

[4] *Lancet* (1872), Oct. 26. 624.

[5] Hamilton Ellis, London, (1950). *Four main lines*. Geo. Allen & Unwin. The first direct Scottish service began in 1840 via Liverpool and Ardrossan. Fourteen hours of the time was sea travel. West Coast trains ran to Kendal, where coaches picked up for Scotland, until 17th Dec., 1846, when the railway reached Carlisle.

[6] *Boston med. surg. J.* (1845), Sept. 24.

[7] *Brit. med. J.* (1894), Oct. 20. 898.

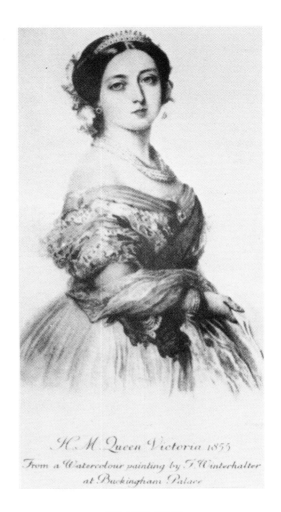

H. M. Queen Victoria 1855
From a Watercolour painting by F. Winterhalter
at Buckingham Palace

PLATE XIII

Scylla—"*We* are having this baby, and *We* are having chloroform."

John Snow's most illustrious patient, as he knew her. Queen Victoria in 1855; age 36. He gave chloroform to her in 1853 and again in 1857. From *The Letters of Queen Victoria*, edited by A. C. Benson and Viscount Esher. 1907. 3 volumes. London: John Murray. Published by authority of H.M. the King.

facing page 77

CHAPTER 4

AN OBSTETRICAL SCYLLA AND CHARYBDIS, OR, VICTORIA AND MR. WAKLEY

V ICTORIA, Queen of Great Britain and Empress of India, is sometimes, quite wrongly, thought to be an uninteresting person, or
even stodgy. I once made this mistake myself. Lytton Strachey,
that debunking biographer, probably had the same idea when he began
to write about her.[1] If so, he very soon found out that he was wrong.
For Victoria refused to be debunked and emerged from his scrutiny as a
person of tremendous vitality. She and her husband, apart altogether
from their exalted position, turned out to be strong characters in their
own right, an impression which is confirmed by my own search through
their writings, many volumes of which I read before dipping into
Strachey's book. The reason for this excursion into Royal biography
will appear later.

Victoria was a woman of abounding energy, to whom nine preg-
nancies were a minor incident in life. Her will was as hard as steel and
she had a most overwhelming personality, in spite of her very small
stature and lack of beauty. In October, 1857, she wrote to the British
Ambassador in Germany about her eldest daughter's marriage:

"The Queen *never* could consent to it (taking place in Berlin) both for
public and private reasons, and the assumption of its being *too much* for a
Prince Royal of Prussia to *come over* to marry *the Princess Royal of Great Britain*
in England is too *absurd*, to say the least. . . . Whatever may be the usual
practice of Prussian Princes, it is not *every* day that one marries the eldest
daughter of the Queen of England. The question therefore must be considered
as settled and closed. . . . "

It was. The marriage took place at the Chapel Royal, St. James's.

A person who could so naturally assume this arrogant and effortless
authority and calmly impose her will upon the head of another dynasty
is not without interest, to say the least of it. And yet she could be very
modest. On one occasion she presented Charles Dickens with a copy of
her own published work.[2] She had written in it, "From the humblest of
writers to one of the greatest." She was diffident about her own attainments, especially as compared to the brilliancy of Albert's, but she was
never modest about the greatness of her position.

She was certainly one of the world's great lovers. Her life with Albert was ideally happy and she worshipped him to adoration. Lytton Strachey says, when he died at the age of forty-two: "With appalling suddenness Victoria had exchanged the serene radiance of happiness for the utter darkness of woe," and this was no exaggeration. The steel-willed autocrat, iron-hard and self sufficient, wrote to her uncle after Albert's death in 1861:

"My own dearest, kindest Father, For as such have I *ever* loved you! The poor fatherless baby of eight months is now the utterly broken-hearted and crushed widow of forty-two! My *life* as a *happy* one is *ended!* The world is gone for *me!* If I must live on . . . it is henceforth for our poor fatherless children—for my unhappy country, which has lost *all* in losing him—and in *only* doing what I know and *feel* he would wish, for he is near me—his spirit will guide and inspire me! But oh! to be cut off in the prime of life—to see our pure, happy, quiet, domestic life, which *alone* enabled me to bear my *much* disliked position, cut off at forty two—when I *had* hoped with such intuitive certainty that God never *would* part us, and would let us grow old together . . . is *too awful*, too cruel! And yet it *must* be for *his* good, his happiness! His purity was too great, his aspiration *too high* for this poor, *miserable* world! His great soul is *now only* enjoying *that* for which it *was* worthy! And I will *not* envy him—only pray that mine may be perfected by it and fit to be with him eternally, for which moment I earnestly long. . . .

Ever your devoted, wretched, child, Victoria R."

Albert himself was perhaps one of the most conscientious men who ever lived. He had a first-class brain, was an expert musician and a tremendous worker. By seven o'clock in the morning he was at his desk, abstracting papers, writing memoranda and doing everything he possibly could to relieve his wife of the burden of State affairs which she had to carry. He is generally thought to have been devoid of a sense of humour, and it is true that he was somewhat stiff, with a formal aloofness which made him a difficult man to know. This was one of the causes of his undeserved unpopularity. But he could tell a story against himself, which is a fair test of that undefinable thing a sense of humour.[3]

"Balmoral is in full splendour. . . . The deer were so polite as to show themselves yesterday . . . in the sacred number of three. Whether from a reverential feeling on our part, or from boundless lack of skill, I know not, but three of us also, to wit, Lord Malmesbury, Col. Phipps and myself, shot . . . and missed them, each of the others twice, and I, as became my rank and station, four times."

On one occasion a man was seen in the street waiting for this resolute pair with a pistol. He escaped in the confusion, so the next day Victoria and her beloved drove past the same spot with the deliberate idea of bringing the matter to a head at once rather than have a continuous threat hanging over them. Their bold plan was successful, but how many of us would have had the cold courage to try it?

The English-speaking world on both sides of the Atlantic owes a great debt to Albert. One of his last actions, at a time when he was feeling very ill indeed (it was the beginning of the attack of typhoid fever which killed him) was to rewrite a provocative diplomatic message which would probably have led to war between the two countries.

In 1853 Mr. Wakley, the fearless and incorruptible watchdog of *The Lancet*, began to hear extraordinary rumours about Her Majesty, rumours which he could hardly believe.[4] Being Mr. Wakley he could not possibly ignore these tales, nor could he keep quiet about them. A leading article appeared:

"A very extraordinary report has obtained general circulation connected with the recent accouchement of her most gracious Majesty Queen Victoria. It has always been understood by the profession that the births of Royal children in all instances have been unattended by any peculiar or untoward circumstances. Intense astonishment, therefore, has been excited throughout the profession by the rumour that her Majesty during her last labour was placed under the influence of chloroform, an agent which has unquestionably caused instantaneous death in a considerable number of cases. Doubts on this subject cannot exist. In several of the fatal examples persons in their usual health expired while the process of inhalation was proceeding, and the deplorable catastrophes were clearly and indisputably referrible (sic) to the poisonous action of the chloroform, and to that cause alone.

"These facts being perfectly well known to the medical world, we could not imagine that anyone had incurred the awful responsibility of advising the administration of chloroform to her Majesty during a perfectly natural labour with a seventh child." (It was, as a matter of fact, the eighth child). "On inquiry, therefore, we were not at all surprised to learn that in her late confinement the Queen was not rendered insensible by chloroform or by any other anæsthetic agent. We state this with feelings of the highest satisfaction. In no case could it be justifiable to administer chloroform in perfectly ordinary labour; but the responsibility of advocating such a proceeding in the case of the Sovereign of these realms would, indeed, be tremendous. Probably some officious meddlers about the Court so far overruled her Majesty's responsible professional advisers as to lead to the pretence of administering chloroform, but we believe the obstetric physicians to whose ability the safety of our illustrious Queen is confided do not sanction the use of chloroform in natural labour. Let it not be supposed that we would undervalue the immense importance of chloroform in surgical operations. We know that an incalculable amount of agony is averted by its employment. On thousands of occasions it has been given without injury, but inasmuch as it has destroyed life in a considerable number of instances, its *unnecessary* inhalation involves, in our opinion, an amount of responsibility which words cannot adequately describe.

"We have felt irresistibly impelled to make the foregoing observations, fearing the consequences of allowing such a rumour respecting a dangerous practice in one of our national palaces to pass unrefuted. Royal examples are followed with extraordinary readiness by a certain class of society in this country."

When I first came across this article I was almost as astonished as Mr. Wakley was, but for a different reason. The first thing to notice is the date—five weeks after the birth of Prince Leopold on April 7th, 1853, so the article obviously refers to this confinement. I checked these details very carefully to make certain that they were correct. This led to further researches into Victoriana, in an effort to explain a conflict of evidence.

The Lancet not only makes it clear that chloroform in normal labour is never justified under any circumstances, but it also states definitely, as a fact, that it was not used. This surprised me very considerably, for I knew that Benjamin Ward Richardson, in his long biographical preface to John Snow's book on chloroform,[5] states categorically that Snow gave chloroform to Her Majesty at this very confinement on the date mentioned above.

"A note in his diary records the event. The inhalation lasted fifty three minutes. The chloroform was given on a handkerchief in fifteen minim doses, and the Queen expressed herself as greatly relieved by the administration. He had previously been consulted on the occasion of the birth of Prince Arthur in 1850, but had not been called in to render his services. . . . On April 14th, 1857, another note in his diary records the fact of the second administration to her Majesty, at the birth of the Princess Beatrice."

That sounds authentic and detailed enough, and it is in flat contradiction to *The Lancet's* leading article. What is the explanation of this discrepancy? Was John Snow a liar, or did Richardson forge the entries in his diary, or was the usually reliable Mr. Wakley mistaken? I think the last of these three alternatives is the correct one, and there is a certain amount of evidence and a good deal of presumption, to support this view, whereas there is none whatever in favour of the other two theories.

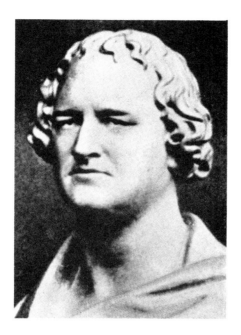

PLATE XIV

Charybdis—"In no case could it be justifiable to administer chloroform in perfectly ordinary labour; but the responsibility of advocating such a proceeding in the case of the Sovereign of these realms would indeed be tremendous."

Thomas Wakley the First, 1795-1862. Founder of *The Lancet*. Editor of *The Lancet*; H.M. Coroner; Member of Parliament. The fearless, implacable, incorruptible watchdog. No money could bribe him. No power on earth could make him keep silent when he thought speech was necessary.

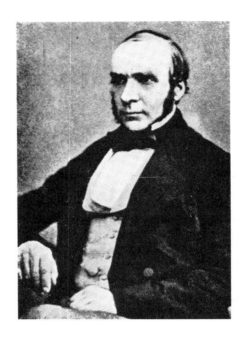

PLATE XV

John Snow, M.D. (1813-1858). From *Disciples of
Aesculapius*, by Sir Benjamin Ward Richardson. 1900.
London: Hutchinson & Co. A duplicate of this picture
is given in *Die Narkose*, by Prof. Dr. H. Killian and Prof.
Dr. H. Weese. Stuttgart: Georg Thieme Verlag. 1954.
First edition, 1934; p. 988. The caption states that Snow
gave chloroform to Queen Victoria at the birth of
Edward VII. The future King was born in 1841, six years
before Simpson announced his discovery.

I say Mr. Wakley was mistaken. What I really mean is that he was deliberately misled.

The obstetrician and the other Royal doctors were in a very perilous dilemma. They were between the devil and the deep sea, so they quibbled. On the one hand was their illustrious patient, who probably demanded chloroform. And when Victoria asked for something she was in the habit of getting it. Her very decisive victory over the German Royal House in the matter of the marriage is distinctly relevant here. If she could bulldoze a crowned head in this effortless way, surely the opposition of a few doctors was child's play to her. After all, only a few years before doctors were expected to use the tradesman's entrance at the back of the house, if indeed they had altogether ceased this habit.

Also a person with a will like hers was not likely to hesitate in making up her mind very definitely on the question of chloroform for her own confinement. No doubt, as *The Lancet* says, the royal doctors were very reluctant to use it. The reasons against it, put forward by Mr. Wakley, were not new to them. They were common knowledge, and a large percentage of doctors agreed with them, at that time. No doubt also the Queen and Albert would listen politely to their objections. After all they had had a lot of practice at listening. Politicians, statesmen, ambassadors, mayors, and deputations of all kinds had been talking at them for years. But I imagine the end of the discussion was in character. "Thank you, gentlemen, for your opinions. *We* are having this baby, and *We* are having chloroform." And another question was settled and closed. I find it quite impossible to imagine the doctors persisting in their refusal in the face of that imperious and inflexible will.

On searching through the relevant parts of the nine volumes of the *Letters of Queen Victoria* I could find no direct reference to this incident.[6] These letters are, of course mainly political, written to her ministers. A few personal and family details are mentioned in those addressed to her relatives, especially those to her uncle the King of the Belgians. But she did not need to ask his advice on an intimate subject like this, which after all concerned nobody but herself and Albert.

On only one occasion—apart from her remarks to John Snow—did she record her opinion of chloroform, and it was entirely favourable. In a letter[7] to Princess Augusta, the mother of the Prince Frederick who married her eldest daughter, also called Victoria, she said, "Vicky appears to feel quite as well and to recover herself just as quickly as I always did. What a blessing she had chloroform! Perhaps without it her strength would have suffered very much."

It must be remembered that, conservative though she was in some ways, in others she was far in advance of her time. In an era when ladies of quality were kept in bed for weeks after their confinements she put into practice—no doubt against strong opposition—the modern idea of getting up early. The Prince Consort himself makes this quite clear in a letter to his stepmother after the birth of the Princess Beatrice (the occasion of the Queen's second anæsthetic): "Victoria is already on the sofa and very well."[8] The birth was on the 14th April and the letter was written on the 19th.

Sidney Lee's biography[9] and Queen Victoria's own book[10] do not mention chloroform at all. There is no particular reason why they should.

So the probability is that the *accoucheur* had to do as he was told, making the best of a bad job by unloading the terrific burden of responsibility on to the competent shoulders of John Snow. He was the acknowledged expert, and had been ever since the beginning of anæsthesia—the only anæsthetist in the kingdom, with the possible exceptions of Clover and Potter.

But imagine the *accoucheur's* horror at the thought of what the formidable Mr. Wakley would say. For he was the other horn of the dilemma, and he was in his own way as inflexible as the Queen herself. Nothing would induce him to be quiet if he had something to say, and he had seen to it that his opinions about chloroform were generally known amongst his professional brethren. He was unbribeable, incorruptible, and utterly fearless. Rank, position and power meant nothing to him, nor was he afraid of the law. Chloroform in normal labour he condemned utterly as a treacherous drug—not knowing yet that it was far safer in labour than in surgery. Mr. Wakley was perhaps even more intimidating than the Queen—if that were possible—for there is no evidence that he ever softened or mellowed at all, whereas Victoria occasionally did. So he had to be pacified by a half-truth—that the Queen was not rendered insensible, which Mr. Wakley interpreted, as he was intended to do, as not having chloroform at all. In actual fact the Queen got her chloroform, given by the best possible man, but she got analgesia only, not anæsthesia—chloroform *à la reine*, in fact. Snow knew quite a lot about anæsthesia by this time, quite enough to use analgesia deliberately. His fifteen minim doses were in fact designed for this purpose, and they did their work well. The Queen herself said so. Mr. Wakley's conjecture that "a pretence of giving chloroform" might have been used was unworthy of his intelligence. Was Victoria the sort of person to be tricked like this?

Technically correct the statement may have been, but as an example of hair-splitting casuistry it takes some beating. For the Editor of *The Lancet* was certainly left with a totally wrong impression. He goes on to pontificate, "In no case could it be justifiable to administer chloroform in normal labour."

Not a very creditable episode, really. One wonders if Victoria and Albert ever got to hear about it. Probably not. It is very unlikely that they had either the time or the inclination to read *The Lancet*. It is equally unlikely that anyone would dare to tell them about it. Anyway John Snow was employed again at a future confinement, so it is quite certain that his work met with the royal approval. But it cost me several weeks of work to ferret out the facts and the background of this affair and to explain the incident in a reasonable way. I can think of no other theory which fits the facts. Whether Mr. Wakley ever found out how he had been diddled is not yet clear. Further researches in later numbers of *The Lancet* should clear up this point.

A detailed search through later volumes, carried out after this chapter was written—I couldn't delay the writing of it because it interested me so much—revealed no further mention of this anæsthesia.

What it did reveal was the fact that I was not quite accurate when I stated that Mr. Wakley never mellowed at all. He, or at any rate his paper, became rather less forthright and less intimidating than before. In 1857 two of his sons were made partners in *The Lancet*. Five years later he died, at the age of sixty-seven. Perhaps he was getting a little tired of fighting, perhaps his sons had a restraining influence. After all, he had corrected so many abuses, defended so many libel actions, exposed so many scandals and advocated so many reforms that the old fire within had probably died down to some extent.

On April 18th, 1857, the year of the family partnership, *The Lancet* reported that "Her Majesty was safely delivered of a Princess . . . on Tuesday last." It was a normal labour, but the report goes on to state, quite calmly, that Dr. Snow began to give chloroform at intervals at 11.30 a.m. This continued for $2\frac{1}{2}$ hours, and "the anæsthetic agent perfectly succeeded in the object desired."

But there was no further comment and no criticism of any kind. I seem to detect the influence of the brothers Wakley here, rather than that of their ruthless and caustic father. In the next week's issue there is a simple and gratified report that Dr. Locock, "who has assisted Her Majesty through so many hours of trial without the occurrence of a single mishap," had been rewarded with a title and had become Sir Charles

Locock, Bart. Sir Charles, then plain Dr. Locock, was appointed physician *accoucheur* to Her Majesty in 1846. She had had four children before this. In 1847 Dr. Robert Ferguson was also appointed to a similar position. So these two were probably responsible for her last five confinements.

Victoria had one other operation during her long life, on Sept. 4th, 1871. Mr. Lister opened an axillary abscess for her, but the reports do not mention any anæsthetic.

Many years later, however, in 1908,[11] Lord Lister, in a long letter to Sir Hector Cameron, gave a condensed history of his antiseptic method. He began by saying that he first treated compound fractures with undiluted carbolic acid in 1865. He then began to use it for abscesses.

"I continued to use a strip of lint as a drain for about five years with perfectly satisfactory results. But in 1871, having opened a very deeply seated acute abscess in the axilla, I found to my surprise on changing the dressing next day that the withdrawal of the lint was followed by escape of thick pus like the original contents. It occurred to me that in that deep and narrow incision, the lint, instead of serving as a drain, might have acted as a plug and so reproduced the conditions present before evacuation."

He goes on to describe in detail how he cut off a piece of rubber tubing from the Richardson's ether spray which had been used at the operation, cut holes in it and attached silk threads to one end. He then soaked it in strong carbolic solution all night and used it for the abscess next morning. He found that there was no further damming up of pus, and the abscess healed in a week. After that he continued to use drainage tubes instead of lint plugs.

Was this patient Victoria? It was the right year, and he goes into such detail that it might well have been the Queen's case. Or it may have been that he detailed it because he thought tubes were a great advance over the old method. We shall never know for certain. But the case does give a hint as to the anæsthesia used. It would certainly be the ether spray.

Much later another little sidelight on this operation was discovered. Sir St. Clair Thomson, one of Lister's house surgeons many years before, gave an address in 1927,[12] revealing many interesting and homely facts about his old chief. In the course of it he said:

"Like all great men he was keen on the importance of small details. In showing us how to bandage a breast he insisted on the point that, in spite of various turns, the bandage was almost sure to slip . . . if the . . . turns of the bandage, above and below . . . the mamma . . . were not prevented from slipping up and down by uniting them with a safety pin. . . . To impress this point upon us he narrated that he had once had to open a simple abscess in the axilla for Queen Victoria. All went well. After one dressing and on arrival at the railway station to travel back to Edinburgh, he suddenly remembered that he had forgotten the important safety pin. He at once drove back to the Castle, and explained his oversight to Her Majesty, and the necessity for rectifying it. Some surgeons, I fear, would have thought first of their own reputation, and would have 'risked' the safety pin."

I have read enough about Victoria to convince me that Lister's frankness and courage in acknowledging his forgetfulness would be appreciated by the patient. Albert would certainly have approved, but, alas, Albert was no longer there.

And so the incident closes. After her second general anæsthetic Victoria had still a few years of perfect happiness with her beloved, before she entered the gloomy and weary thirty-nine years of loneliness and sorrow. Only as death approached did the shadows lighten, at the joyous prospect of reunion. When she was dead there was to be no black upon her, for the first time for four long decades. So, at eighty-one, she was buried with her wedding veil in her coffin.

Dr. Locock had the vastly increased professional prestige of his baronetcy, Mr. Wakley, though still alive, lay dormant like an extinct volcano, and Dr. Snow, being an anæsthetist, naturally got nothing out of it at all.

REFERENCES

[1] Lytton Strachey (1921). *Queen Victoria.* (310 pp.). London. Chatto and Windus.

[2] Queen Victoria (1868). *Leaves from the Journal of our life in the Highlands.* (315 pp.). Smith, Elder and Co.

[3] Theodore Martin. *Life of the Prince Consort.* 5 volumes. Vol. 2. 462. Letter from the Prince to the Dowager Duchess of Coburg. London. Smith, Elder and Co.

[4] *Lancet* (1853), May 14. 453.

[5] John Snow (1858). *On Chloroform and other anæsthetics.* 423 pp. London. John Churchill.

[6] *Letters of Queen Victoria* (1907). 9 volumes. London. John Murray.

[7] *Further Letters of Queen Victoria* (1938). 278 pp.; 105. Edited by Hector Bolitho. London. Thornton Butterworth.

[8] Theodore Martin (1879). *Life of the Prince Consort.*

[9] Sidney Lee (1903). *Queen Victoria* 575 pp. Smith, Elder.

[10] Queen Victoria (1868). *Leaves from the Journal of our life in the Highlands.* 315 pp. Smith, Elder.

[11] *Lancet* (1908), June 27. 1815.

[12] *Lancet* (1927), April 9. 77. Sir St. Clair Thomson. One of Lister's ex-house surgeons.

CHAPTER 5

CURARE, OR, THE SQUIRE OF WALTON

SIR WALTER RALEGH (for that was the way he preferred to spell his name) was born in 1552 in Devonshire. He went to Oriel College, Oxford, and then became a soldier and a sailor, both General and Admiral. He was a treasure hunter and a pirate, a courtier, a poet, an author and a historian. He was the first man to introduce potatoes and tobacco to the Western world. His varied and colourful career ended suddenly when he was beheaded on 29th October, 1618.

In 1595 he wrote:[1]

"There was nothing whereof I was more curious, than to finde out the true remedies of these poisoned arrowes, for besides the mortalitie of the wound they make, the partie shot indureth the most insufferable torment in the world, and abideth a most vgly and lamentable death, sometimes dying starke mad, sometimes their bowels breaking out of their bellies, and are presently discolored, as black as pitch, and so vnsauery, as no man can endure to cure, or to attend them; And it is more strange to know, that in all this time there was never Spaniard, either by gift or torment that could attaine to the true knowledge of the cure, although they have martyred and put to inuented torture I know not how many of them. But euery one of these Indians know it not, no not one among thousands, but their soothsaiers and priests, who do conceale it, and only teach it but from the father to the sonne.

"Those medicines which are vulgar, and serue for the ordinarie poison, are made of the iuce of a roote called Tupara: the same also quencheth maruellously the heate of burning feauers, and healeth inward wounds, and broken veines, that bleed within the body. But I was more beholding to the Guianians than any other, for Antonio de Berreo told me that he could neuer attaine to the knowledge thereof, and yet they taught me the best way of healing as wel thereof, as of al other poisons. Some of the Spaniards have been cured in ordinary wounds, of the common poisoned arrowes with the iuce of garlike: but this is a generall rule for all men that shall hereafter trauell the Indies where poisoned arrowes are vsed, that they must abstain from drinke, for if they take any licor into their body, I say, if they drink before the wound be dressed, or soone upon it, there is no way with them but present death."

The editor of the Hakluyt Society edition, Sir Robert Schomburgk, has a long footnote to Ralegh's remarks:

THE
DISCOVERIE
OF THE LARGE,
RICH AND BEWTIFVL
EMPIRE OF Gviana, WITH
a relation of the Great and Golden City
of Manoa *(which the spaniards call* El
Dorado*)* And the prouinces of *Emeria,
Arromaia, Amapaia* and other Countries, with their riuers, ad-
ioyning.

Performed in the yeare 1595. by Sir
W. Ralegh, Knight, Captaine of her
Maiesties Guard, Lo. Warden
of the Stanneries, and her High-
nesse Lieutenant generall
of the Countie of
Cornewall.

Jmprinted at London by Robert Robinson
1596.

Fig. 17

"The mystery respecting the arrow-poison of the Indians, although not entirely cleared up, is in a great measure removed. Neither snakes' teeth nor stinging ants form the active principle, but the juice of a plant which we have described as *Strychnos toxifera*. . . . This plant is only known to grow in three or four situations in Guiana, and is in its habit a ligneous twiner or bushrope (which kinds of plants are called in the French colonies Liane, and by the Spaniards Bejuco). The Indians of the Macusi tribe are the best manufacturers of the poison, which is entirely composed of the juice of plants. Previous travellers during the present century in Guiana never saw it prepared, nor did they see the plant growing of which it is made; and the accounts which they have given us of its preparation were perhaps imposed upon them by the Carabisis, but rest surely not upon personal experience, as they are so very erroneous. The Macusis call the plant Urari-yè, the poison itself Urari (read ourahree) which the Carabisi, who constantly interchange the r and l, have corrupted into Urali and Ulari, of which Wurali has been made. The Caribs are not able to prepare the poison, and purchase it from the Macusis. It is surprising to us why a spurious name should have been substituted in England for the true one, since we find the proper name of the poison mentioned already by Keymis in Hakluyt (vol. III, p. 687) in a table of names and rivers, &c., where under the head of poisoned herbs occurs the plant 'Ourari'. The author of these notes has given an unadorned account of the mode of preparing the poison in the *Annals of Natural History*, vol. VII, p. 407, and he has prepared it himself, by concentrating merely the infusion from the bark of the plant (*Stychnos toxifera*) which had been collected in his presence. It killed a fowl in twenty seven minutes, although not sufficiently concentrated. Well prepared poison, which is of a dark colour, shows its effects in the space of a minute, and kills a fowl in five minutes. Its effect is more or less sudden upon different animals, and the Indians say that monkeys and jaguars are more easily killed with it than any other animals. We have been assured repeatedly by the Indians that there is no remedy against the Urari if it be good—salt and sugar are both considered antidotes against weak poison, but avail nothing where the Urari is strong. It has been related to us that, when wounded in wars, and salt is not to be had, the Indians resort to urine. The thirst which follows is described as almost intolerable, and certain death ensues if the thirst is quenched with water; the more the wounded person drinks, the greater becomes his thirst. Ralegh's relation is therefore perfectly correct in this respect. It has not been possible as yet to procure a perfect analysis of the Urari. The agent which destroys the vital powers in so short a period appears to be a new principle, hitherto unknown to chemists. Numerous experiments have recently been made with it in Berlin."

Sir Robert himself investigated the famous arrow poison and wrote a twenty page article about it, as he mentioned in his footnote.[2]

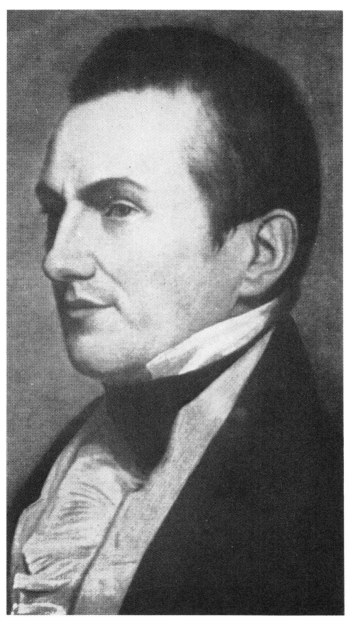

PLATE XVI

Charles Waterton, the Squire of Walton Hall. Philip Gosse. London, 1940: Cassell & Co. From the National Portrait Gallery.

facing page 88

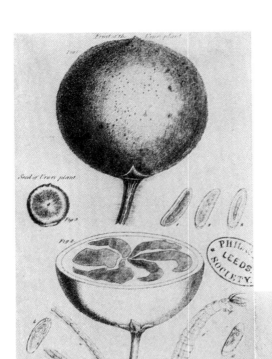

PLATE XVII

Sir Robert Schomburgk.
Annals of Natural History.
1841. Vol. VII. Fruit
and flower of the Urari
plant.

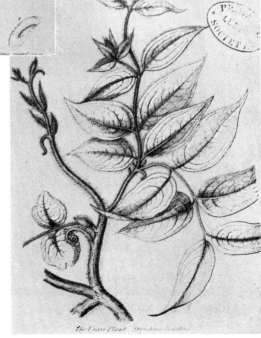

In the early nineteenth century, three hundred and seventeen years after Ralegh's cursory investigations, and in the same year in which the frostbitten remnants of Napoleon's Grand Army struggled back from Moscow, a charming and eccentric individual set out for South America on a voyage of exploration, one of the objects being to collect specimens of curare.

His name was Charles Waterton, and he is mentioned in the footnotes to almost every paper written on this subject. But he is so interesting a character that he deserves to be rescued from this forgotten limbo of small print.

He lived at Walton Hall, three miles south of Wakefield, only about ten miles away from my home. So I went there and photographed his house, which has altered very little since Dr. Hobson's engraving of it was published ninety years ago. It is a large house standing on an island in a lake, surrounded by a park of surprising beauty. The country round is rather grim. Coal mines, factories, and the ugliness of an industrial area have scarred it badly, but no trace of this man-made chaos is visible from the house or in the park. The Squires of Walton have long since departed and the Hall is now a Maternity Home belonging to the Wakefield Corporation. Dr. Richard Hobson of Leeds wrote a book about the Squire in 1867;[3] he also was impressed by the character of this eccentric and extraordinary man.

The Watertons had lived at Walton Hall for centuries. Tradition has it that the Hall was unsuccessfully besieged by Oliver Cromwell, and evidence of the truth of this was found when a swivel cannon was dredged from the lake in 1857 in the spot predicted by the legend. The Squire of the time was away, probably on field service with the Royalist Army, and his wife was in charge of the defence against the formidable dictator. Cromwell, though he was not able to capture the Hall with its magnificent natural moat, took away all the horses when he raised the siege, so the undaunted Mrs. Waterton proudly yoked six oxen to her carriage there-after. Dr. Hobson says that many bullets remain embedded in one of the doors.

Squire Waterton made the three hundred acre park into a bird sanctuary, and listed 119 different species seen in it. He was an enthusiastic ornithologist, an expert taxidermist and a naturalist in the widest sense of the word. Shooting in the park was forbidden and no boats were allowed on the lake from September to May. He was a Catholic and very often used to supply the Friday's fish by shooting them in the lake with a bow and arrow, which would not disturb his birds.

After his wife died he never went to bed for thirty years, but slept on the floor with a wooden pillow. He got up—not surprisingly—at 3.30 a.m. He was a teetotaller and was in the habit of wearing old and dilapidated clothes. On one occasion he was visiting a neighbouring colonel and was shown into the servants' hall by mistake. He made a practice of bleeding himself frequently and profusely. On another occasion he made himself a pair of wings and was only dissuaded with difficulty from launching himself from the roof of a building to try them out. At the age of 81 he could stand in the upper branches of a tree or on top of a high wall without fear of falling. He died on May 27th, 1865, aged 82.

His first voyage to South America was in 1812.[4] The strongest *wourali* poison, he stated, was made by the Macoushi tribe. It was important that the arrows should be kept dry. He describes the blowpipe and darts and the bows and arrows used. The arrows were made with detachable poisoned tips and—an important point—protecting caps for the sharp ends. A wild hog, shot in the cheek by one of these arrows, was found dead 170 paces away and was eaten for supper. A sloth died in ten minutes, a large ox in twenty-five minutes. The antidotes recommended by the Indians were—holding the animal up to the mouth in water and the giving of sugar cane juice, but Waterton found these ineffectual.

"It is supposed to affect the nervous system, and thus destroy the vital functions; it is also said to be perfectly harmless, provided it does not touch the blood. However, this is certain, when a sufficient quantity of it enters the blood, death is the inevitable consequence; but there is no alteration in the colour of the blood, and both the blood and the flesh may be eaten with safety. . . . A vine grows in these wilds, which is called *wourali*. It is from this that the poison takes its name, and it is the principal ingredient. When he has procured enough of this, he digs up a root of a very bitter taste, ties them together, and then looks about for two kinds of bulbous plants, which contain a green and glutinous juice. He fills a little quake, which he carries on his back, with the stalks of these; and lastly, ranges up and down till he finds two species of ants. One of them is very large and black, and so venomous, that its sting produces a fever; it is most commonly to be met with on the ground. The other is a little red ant, which stings like a nettle, and generally has its nest under the leaf of a shrub. A quantity of the strongest Indian pepper is used; but this he has already planted round his hut. The pounded fangs of the Labarri snake, and those of the Counacouchi, are likewise added."

Waterton then describes the infusion and its concentration by boiling. It is then put in a pot and kept dry. Women and girls are not allowed to witness the making of it, which must be carried out fasting, in a new pot. Other elements of magic enter into the ceremony. Waterton doubted whether all the ingredients are necessary, but was not sure.

"It is supposed by some, that wind introduced into the lungs by a small pair of bellows, would revive the poisoned patient, provided the operation be continued for a sufficient length of time. It may be so. . . ." He also recommended a tight ligature and excision of the wound by the knife. On returning to England further experiments were carried out.

"An ass was inoculated with it, and died in twelve minutes. The poison was inserted into the leg of another, round which a bandage had been previously tied a little above the place where the *wourali* was introduced. He walked about as usual, and ate his food as though all were right. After an hour had elapsed, the bandage was untied, and ten minutes after death overtook him.

"A she-ass received the *wourali* poison in the shoulder, and died apparently in ten minutes. An incision was then made in its windpipe, and through it the lungs were regularly inflated for two hours with a pair of bellows. Suspended animation returned. . . ."

On stopping the inflation she "sunk once more in apparent death." Controlled respiration was continued for another two hours and recovery took place. The donkey was sent to Walton Hall, named Wouralia, and ended her days in peace. The Squire would be interested to see his method in constant use by anæsthetists today, possibly even in his own house in its capacity as a Maternity Home.

Dr. Hobson describes in his book how he invited forty doctors to his house in Leeds on one occasion, when a comparative test was to be made between the *Wourali* poison and that of the rattlesnake. Mr. Waterton, as the only *Wourali* expert, was also invited. Twenty-eight snakes were available, more than ready to take their part in the experiment, and pigeons and rabbits were provided as victims. Everything was organised beautifully, but the proceedings came to a standstill owing to one small point which had been overlooked. No one was willing to hold the rabbits inside the cages, or even to go anywhere near the snakes at all.

The whole experimental programme looked like being a complete wash-out when Mr. Waterton stepped forward and saved the situation from utter failure. He asked for absolute silence and went from cage to cage, catching each rattlesnake by the neck with one hand and presenting the victim to it with the other.

CHARLES WATERTON:

HIS

HOME, HABITS, AND HANDIWORK.

REMINISCENCES OF AN INTIMATE AND MOST CONFIDING PERSONAL
ASSOCIATION FOR NEARLY THIRTY YEARS.

BY

RICHARD HOBSON, M.D., Cantab.,

LEEDS

SECOND EDITION
CONTAINING A CONSIDERABLE AMOUNT OF ADDITIONAL MATTER.

WITH SIXTEEN ILLUSTRATIONS
ENGRAVED FROM PHOTOGRAPHS OBTAINED WITHIN THE GROUNDS AT WALTON HALL,
BY SAMUEL SMITH AND THE LATE W LYNDON SMITH, FSQRS

"MULTIS ILLE BONIS FLEBILIS OCCIDIT.
NULLI FLEBILIOR QUAM" MIHI

"He died lamented by many good men,
By none more lamented than" by me.

LONDON

WHITTAKER & Co   SIMPKIN. MARSHALL, & Co.

LEEDS   JOHN SMITH, AND H W WALKER

MDCCCLXVIL

FIG. 18
Dr. Richard Hobson of Leeds wrote a book about the Squire in 1867.

He calmly continued to do this with perfect success in every case except one. Here the cage-opener bungled the job and a large and extremely disgruntled snake very nearly escaped. Everybody panicked except Mr. Waterton. "In the sudden determination to beat a hasty retreat at every hazard, nearly all fled from their supposedly perilous position, and several not only rushed downstairs, but even into the street without their hats"—only the very gravest emergency could cause a respectable nineteenth century doctor to go into the street without his top hat!

Mr. Waterton's theory was that snakes only attack when provoked, and that he gave them no provocation until he had them firmly and harmlessly held by the neck. The theory worked well in practice, but it is not every man who would care to try it. But what was a mere snake to a man who had ridden astride on a live crocodile? This exploit he relates in his own book, with pictures and a description of the precautions taken.

"I had no fear, because I knew it was impossible that the hook . . . could be returned through the mouth, and having made it myself, I had carefully ascertained that there was no flaw in it, and had also tested the strength of the rope. You may rely upon it that I had made all secure for the sake of number one. . . . "

If one must ride on a live crocodile it is certainly just as well to be sure of these points.

The Squire believed that the *Wourali* poison would cure hydrophobia, and several times he was sent for in order to put his theories into practice, but the patients all died before he got there.

Work on curare after Waterton's time became much less exciting. It entirely lacks the dramatic touch of the master hand, though Schomburgk's twenty-page article is not without interest. [5] He says that much mystery and legend had accumulated on this subject. It is said

"that the pernicious exhalations which arise from the pots cause the old women to perish who are chosen to watch over this operation; finally, that these vegetable juices never are considered as sufficiently concentrated till a few drops produce at a distance a repulsive action on the blood. An Indian wounds himself slightly, and a dart dipped in the liquid curare is held near the wound; if it makes the blood return to the vessels without having been brought in contact with them, the poison is judged to be sufficiently concentrated." (Father Gumilla).

WANDERINGS

IN

SOUTH AMERICA,

THE

NORTH-WEST OF THE UNITED STATES,

And the Antilles,

IN THE YEARS 1812, 1816, 1820, & 1824.

WITH ORIGINAL

INSTRUCTIONS FOR THE PERFECT PRESERVATION OF BIRDS, &c.

FOR CABINETS OF NATURAL HISTORY.

BY CHARLES WATERTON, ESQ.

SECOND EDITION.

LONDON:

PRINTED FOR

B. FELLOWES, (SUCCESSOR TO Mr. MAWMAN,)

LUDGATE STREET

1828.

FIG. 19

Charles Waterton's first voyage to South America was in 1812.

J. J. Hartzinck was

"informed that, in order to try whether the poison be good, a poisoned arrow is shot into a young tree; if the tree shed its leaves in the course of three days the poison is considered strong enough. He observes further, that in the last rebellion of the negroes in Berbice, a woman who carried her child on her back was shot with a poisoned arrow, and though the child was not wounded, it began to swell, and died a short time after."

Schomburgk thinks that Waterton's description did not rest on personal experience. He wanted to find out for himself whether the other ingredients (ants, snakes' fangs, etc.) were really necessary. He found out that the plant grew on the Conocon or Canuku Mountains. "After I had engaged some guides, I started, accompanied by Lieut. Haining of the 65th Regiment, in the morning of the 25th of December, in search of the mysterious plant. . . ." It was rough going, and Schomburgk takes two pages to describe the journey, but eventually he saw the Urari growing among the trees. It was not in flower but was bearing fruit. He named it *Strychnos toxifera,* and devotes two pages to its botanical description. It is a ligneous twiner which winds itself round the neighbouring trees.

"The Wapisianas and Macusis are generally acknowledged to be the best manufacturers of the poison. . . . It is only the bark of the woody parts and its alburnum which are considered to possess the poisonous principle in the highest degree. The stem of the plant is therefore cut into pieces about three feet in length, of which the bark is stripped, and after having been pounded it is steeped in water, for which purpose a new earthen vessel is used; here they allow it to remain for some time, well covered, until the water is of a yellowish colour, when it is filtered through a funnel-shaped matappa lined with plantain-leaves. Several other plants have been meanwhile procured, and after their juice has been extracted in a similar manner, this extract is kept ready to be added to the former at the moment it has been concentrated on a slow fire to the consistency of a syrup. The addition of that juice gives a darker colour to the Urari, which, from the time of its becoming concentrated, has the appearance of tar; it is now put into small calabashes, which are covered with leaves to prevent the poison from coming in immediate contact with the air. The Indians pretend, that if it be well preserved it will keep its strength for a couple of years. . . . After that juice has been added to it, the Indian buries the calabash with the poison for a day or two under ground. . . ."

This was the account given to Schomburgk, but people would not believe it. The stories of snakes' teeth and stinging ants had taken too strong a hold. In 1837 he returned to Guiana and bribed an Indian to prepare the stuff in his presence. He went with the Indian to gather the plant, but again failed to find it in blossom. On returning the Indian was apparently forbidden by a chief to carry out his promise, so Schomburgk himself tried to make it. He took two pounds of the bark shavings and macerated them in a gallon of water for twenty-four hours. Half of it was filtered off and boiled, adding from time to time more of the infusion. After it had reached a thin, syrupy consistency two arrows were poisoned with it and two fowls wounded. The first died in 27 minutes, the second in twenty-eight. The boiling had lasted seven hours, while the Indians boiled it for two days, so it was evidently not concentrated enough. But Schomburgk had proved his point to his own satisfaction. Two years later he saw the process carried out by the Indians, but for some reason or other, instead of describing what he saw, he quotes a long description by the Rev. Thomas Yond, a missionary, who spells it Urary —yet another variant. The operator insisted on lighting his fire with his own tinder box and would not make use of a fire which was already available. His recipe was Urary bark 2 lb., Arimarn bark $\frac{1}{4}$ lb., Tarireng $\frac{1}{4}$ lb., Yakkee $\frac{1}{4}$ lb., Wokarimo $\frac{1}{4}$ lb., Taruemu $\frac{1}{2}$ oz., Muramu, a root $1\frac{1}{4}$ lb., Manuca bark, 4 small pieces. All these were plants.

Two days were occupied in boiling these, in two separate consignments, as the pot was too small to contain the whole quantity. A gallon and a half of liquid was finally reduced to about a quart, which was then filtered and allowed to stand in the sun in shallow plates for about two days. Eventually the whole was reduced to about half a pint in volume. The Indians then tried it on three lizards, which died in a few minutes. A rat then died before it could move ten feet. A fowl then died very quickly, and was eaten for Yond's dinner. This Indian did not use ants or snakes' teeth at all. He abstained from meat, requested Yond not to eat or drink sugar and would not go to chapel that Sunday.

Schomburgk saw a deer shot with a poisoned arrow. It died before it had covered forty yards. He found that the Indians were correct in saying that it kept well. He killed a rabbit in four or five minutes with a specimen which he knew to be fifteen months old.

Mr. Sewell, a veterinary surgeon, tried Urari in the treatment of tetanus in horses. He argued that "if a horse in tetanus were destroyed by poison, which acts by suppressing nervous power, and life were then to be restored by artificial respiration, the nervous system, on re-animation taking place, might possibly be free of the original morbid irritation." A horse whose mouth was tightly closed owing to tetanus was inoculated with Urari and in ten minutes apparently died. Artificial respiration

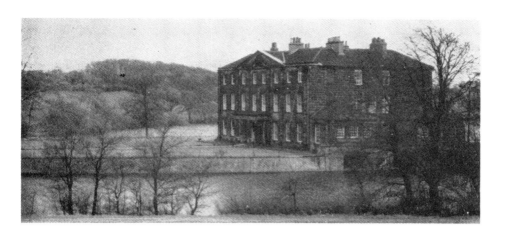

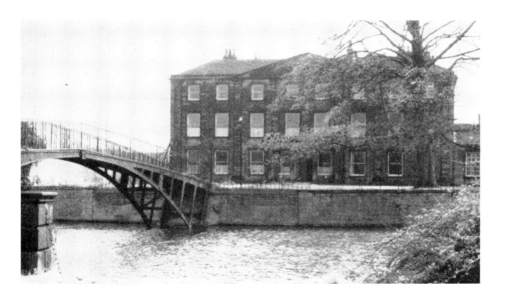

PLATE XVIII

Squire Waterton lived at Walton Hall, near Wakefield.
I went there and photographed his house.

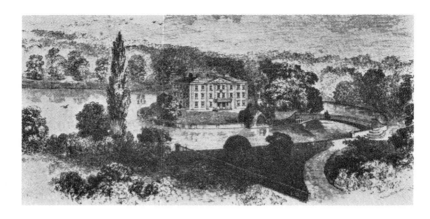

PLATE XIX

It has altered very little since Dr. Hobson's engraving of it was published
ninety years ago.

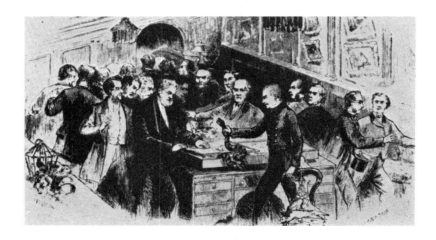

PLATE XX

Twenty-eight snakes were available at Dr. Hobson's house,
more than ready to take their part in the experiments.

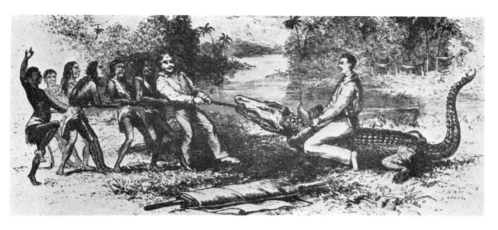

PLATE XXI

What was a mere snake to a man who had ridden astride
on a live crocodile?

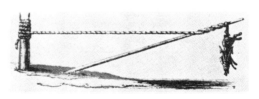

PLATE XXIII

. . and I had also tested the
strength of the rope.

PLATE XXII

Having made it my-
self I had carefully
ascertained that
there was no flaw in
the hook. . . .

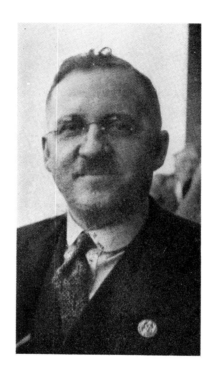

PLATE XXIV

Harold Griffith of Montreal. Taken by
the author in 1936, in Philadelphia, Pa.
He introduced curare into modern
practice in 1942.

was kept up for four hours, when the horse got up and ate hay and corn. Next day he died of over-distension of the stomach, without any return of the tetanic spasm.

It was also proposed to use it in hydrophobia. Squire Waterton, on one occasion was asked to go to Nottingham to treat Inspector Phelps, but unfortunately the patient died before he got there. Schomburgk took Urari internally for tertian ague in the absence of quinine, but stopped it when he realised the danger of an excoriation of the tongue or throat. He says that a Carib chief confirmed Sir Walter Ralegh's statement about the intolerable thirst which follows a wound. He had no faith in sugar cane juice as an antidote, which he had tried unsuccessfully.

Spencer Wells reported three cases of tetanus in which woorara was used in 1859.[6] Ten years later Demme had treated 22 cases with 8 recoveries and Busch 11 cases, of which 6 recovered.[7] Goldman states that F. P. de Caux used curare in 1928 to obtain muscular relaxation under nitrous oxide and oxygen anæsthesia.[8] Certainly de Caux was a keen believer in the use of gas oxygen by McKesson's technique.

Ranyard West published experimental work on curare in man in 1932,[9] and again in 1935.[10] He found that it had a differential action, that tetany in dogs could be abolished by half the dose required to produce paresis. An extract was made from some 30 year old curare and given hypodermically to thirty patients. The results in two cases of epilepsy were negative, but in rigidity due to pyramidal lesions and in Parkinsonism there was a reduction in rigidity. This rigidity-reducing or 'lissive' action was not present in all samples. Curare is a mixture of watery extracts of a number of poisonous plants, differing in different areas. Some produce convulsions, some do not. The constant element is *Strychnos toxifera*. The action of this variable and unstandardised substance was so irregular and so unreliable that West's articles are very confusing. He himself finally concluded, "I think the therapeutic uses of curarine will remain very limited." Seven years later Griffiths of Montreal brought it into general use.

REFERENCES

1 *The Discoverie of the large, rich and bewtiful Empire of Guiana . . . Performed in the yeare* 1595, *by Sir W. Ralegh, Knight, Captaine of her Maiestie's Guard, Lo. Warden of the Stannaries, and her Highneffe Lieutenant general of the Countie of Cornewall.* Imprinted at London by Robert Robinson, 1596. Reprinted for the Hakluyt Society, London, 1868.

2 *Ann. Nat. Hist.* (1841). Vol. VII. 407.

3 Dr. Richard Hobson (1867). *Charles Waterton; his home, habits and handiwork.* 375 pp. London. Simpkin, Marshall and Co.

4 Charles Waterton (1828). *Wanderings in South America.* 2nd edition. 341 pp. (pp. 51-75 and p. 83). London. B. Fellowes.

5 *Ann. Nat. Hist.* (1841). Vol. VII. 407. On the Urari, the arrow poison of the Indians of Guiana; with a description of the plant from which it is extracted.

6 *Proc. R. med.-chir. Soc.* (1859). (Lond.). 3. Reference not checked.

7 *Med. Tms. Gaz.* (1869). May 1. 474.

8 Victor Goldman (1941) *Aids to Anæsthesia.* 2nd ed., 1954.

9 *Proc. R. Soc. med.* (1932). 1107. 9 page article

10 *Proc. R. Soc. med.* (1935). 565. 13½ page article.

CHAPTER 6

STUPIDITIES

Gegen die Dummheit kämpfen die Götter selbst vergebens.
(Against stupidity the gods themselves battle in vain.)

—GOETHE.

IT was Sydney Smith, the Victorian wit, who said that proper attention would never be given to the prevention of railway accidents until a Bishop was killed in one of them. Even Sodor and Man would do, he added hopefully. (The Bishop of Sodor and Man is the Bishop of the Isle of Man. Sodor is apparently a sort of myth, with no real existence. This Bishop, no doubt for some historical reason, is the only one on the episcopal list who can never sit in the House of Lords. Don't ask me why. This is not an ecclesiastical history.)

The Lancet[1] comments on a chloroform death at Epsom in a somewhat similar way. The chloroform was given by a druggist for the extraction of a tooth. This operation in itself, says the article, is not attended by any danger at all, therefore no dentist, still less a druggist, has any right to risk the life of a patient during an extraction by using chloroform.

"This time it was a servant girl who was sacrificed; the next time it may be a duchess." Sure enough there was not long to wait before the prophecy came, at any rate partially, true. In those days practically every week's issue carried reports of one or more chloroform deaths.

Eight weeks later[2] "a lady of wealth and influence at Barnes" enacted the unenviable role of Sodor and Man. True, she was not a duchess, but —she was by no means a servant girl. Mr. Lawrence was the surgeon, and Holmes Coote gave the anæsthetic—the two surgeons of St. Bartholomew's Hospital who had used diluted chloroform (as chloric ether) several months before Simpson's first announcement.

This time, of course, they used the undiluted drug. It was ten years later than their first trials. It was given on a handkerchief, the very method which *The Lancet* had been condemning publicly for months. Holmes Coote gave evidence at the inquest that he had taken every precaution by gradually applying it (chloroform) to the system. The verdict was, of course, accidental death. "Every precaution," comments *The Lancet*, with something of a return to its old pontifical severity (I think Mr. Wakley senior must have written this)—"is a phrase which can only be interpreted according to the knowledge and opinion of the person who employs it. In this case . . . the most important precaution was omitted."

Once more *The Lancet* patiently and wearily repeats Snow's dictum that 5% of vapour is the maximum which can be inhaled safely; and that the rag and bottle method cannot guarantee any constant strength at all. Not only is the strength unknown, but it can, and does, fluctuate within very wide limits.

Four years earlier[3] *The Lancet* had said, "Week after week deaths by chloroform are recorded, until at length these events have become so common that they scarcely attract attention. This cannot and must not be. . . ."

Again,[4] after deaths at Epsom and Dorking:
"this dangerous but most blessed vapour should never be administered in uncontrolled quantity and strength upon a napkin. Dr. Snow has left us an instrument which bears his name, by which the quantity administered can be most accurately regulated and registered, and the dilution of the vapour ensured up to any point. But, on the other hand, when chloroform is administered upon a napkin or upon a handkerchief, its dilution cannot be controlled. At one breath it is swallowed almost pure, and at the next greatly admixed with air. . . . "

A little later[5] Wm. Hooper Attree suggested that it be made compulsory by law to have two anæsthetists at every case, one to give chloroform by Snow's apparatus, the other to watch the pulse.

Lawrence and Coote, at any rate, had the fact forcibly impressed upon them by the sudden death of this private patient, that chloroform was no respecter of persons or incomes, that ladies of wealth and influence were no more immune from chloroform death than mere servant girls, and that surgeons of standing and renown could have the same tragic accidents as tooth-pulling druggists.

But the idea that anyone could give an anæsthetic was unconscionably slow in dying. People would not admit that any knowledge, training, experience or skill was required, despite the constant and steady stream of reports of chloroform deaths. Some writers, otherwise intelligent, ignored the evidence and said that the risk was trivial. Lauder Brunton, a physiologist of some repute, stated in 1895:

"the dread of pain has of late years been replaced by a dread of the anæsthetic which would relieve it, and many people will now suffer the short, but extremely severe pain caused by the extraction of a tooth rather than run the trivial risk of using an anæsthetic."

The general public had, at any rate, sufficient sense to realise that, although the percentage of deaths might be statistically and numerically small, each fatality was 100% dead, a fact which appears to have escaped the attention of the physiologist.

Sir Walter Simpson was surprised, in 1889, that doctors wasted time discussing the comparative safety of different anæsthetics, as if it was of any practical importance. "Statistically speaking, the percentage of deaths is so small as to be practically nil." *The Lancet* deals with this astounding statement with the same sound commonsense as the general public.

Even if statistics were of any value, as applied to the individual, there remained the difficulty of obtaining them. Woolly-minded individuals rushed into print, proclaiming their views without the slightest idea how many cases they had seen. W. Martin Coates[6] is a fair example of this. "Although I have during these 24 years never been prevented from administering it by extreme old age or infancy, by chronically diseased heart, lungs or kidney, I have not had a death by chloroform. Considering that I have been surgeon to the Salisbury Infirmary during all these years, and have had during that period a numerous clientèle, this evidence will, I trust, be considered important."

It is a far cry from 'a numerous clientèle' to the χ^2 mysteries of today.

In the same year *The Lancet*, referring to the steady stream of deaths reported in its columns, said,

"the responsibilities of the profession on this count are without limit. It . . . brought in the agent which caused the deaths; on its recommendation the general public accepted the agent, and by and through its voice declared the anæsthetic beneficent and its introducers the greatest benefactors of the human race. Is all this a delusion? . . . from the very first days when it was itself brought in, chloroform has brought in death. Within ten weeks of its discovery as an anæsthetic, and long before it had come into general use, it caused the death of a girl fifteen years of age in this country . . . one death in 2500 . . . is in fact a large mortality. Applied to any other human act, it were an intolerable evil."

Anæsthetists were satirical about it. T. D. Luke, an Edinburgh anæsthetist, wrote in 1908:

"Some surgeons say that there is one anæsthetic and that is chloroform. Chloroform may be given anyhow, anywhere, by anyone. If the patient shows signs of impending dissolution he is said to take the chloroform badly. If he does not he takes it well. If he dies it is an act of God. An anæsthetist is defined as a latter-day nuisance, of no use to the surgeon and a curse to the G.P. There is no more need for the anæsthetist than for a hypodermic injectionist or other poisonist."

This is really a summary—and not an unfair one, in spite of its bitter sarcasm—of Syme's principles, which evidently still persisted right into the twentieth century.

Dudley Buxton, about the same time, commented that giving an anæsthetic for an unqualified person was the deadly sin of 'covering,' which carried the inevitable penalty of being struck off the Register. What was the difference between this and handing over the anæsthetic to an unqualified person, a thing which was done every day without the slightest risk of any penalty at all?

Some brought forward arguments which were simply not true. John Horsfall of Leeds attacked Joy Jeffries, a great American protagonist of ether, who was mainly responsible for its renaissance in England. Jeffries had urged "the fearfully increasing fatality of chloroform" as a reason for using ether. Horsfall stated that this was a great exaggeration. "In this island alone chloroform is given every day to at least 1,500 to 2,000 individuals, or say to about 600,000 per annum. And how rarely do we hear of a death *under* it; *from* it almost never."

It is quite obvious that Mr. Horsfall was not a reader of *The Lancet*. Alexander Wilson, the first Manchester anæsthetist, quickly punctured this balloon,[7] by pointing out that in the medical journals for the last ten years there were reported at least 120 deaths from chloroform. In at least forty-nine the patients were in good health and the operation was trivial. In 59 cases death occurred before the operation was begun.

J. F. W. Silk pleaded for tuition in anæsthesia in 1892. He stated that there was no systematic instruction in anæsthesia in Scotland, Ireland or the provinces. Any anæsthetists there were in these areas were functional only and not academic. Things were a little better in London, he admitted, but he said that the death rate was treated far too lightly. The deaths from anæsthetics in England alone in the ten years 1881-1890 were 327, 287 or 87·7% of them being registered as due to chloroform.

In 1901 the Society of Anæsthetists pointed out to the General Medical Council that (*a*) there was no compulsory training in anæsthesia in any hospital or teaching centre in the whole of Great Britain and Ireland; (*b*) that there was no examination in this subject; (*c*) that the giving of an anæsthetic involves risk to life; (*d*) that every doctor is liable to be called upon to give one; (e) that in view of the importance of the subject compulsory instruction should be insisted upon.

The Education Committee of the Council replied with two conflicting and incompatible statements. They stated that they fully appreciated the importance of proper teaching in the subject of anæsthesia, but they were of opinion that it is not expedient for it to be compulsorily included in the medical curriculum.

The next year Nicol Jarvie[8] made some acid but perfectly legitimate comments upon Dr. Heron Watson, who took part in the General Medical Council's discussion on the subject. (Sir Patrick Heron Watson was born on Jan. 5, 1832. He qualified in 1853 and served in the Crimean War. He became surgeon to the Edinburgh Royal Infirmary and was knighted in 1903. He was a brilliant surgeon, but poor at antiseptic details. He died Dec. 21, 1907.) Dr. Watson, as he then was, had said that the subject was taught in Scottish Universities, that nurses and dressers were taught the use of chloroform in Scottish Hospitals and Infirmaries, and that there were no accidents from anæsthesia in these institutions.

Jarvie said that the 'teaching' was confined to one lecture, by a surgeon, which was often omitted altogether. Clinically the students, before they knew any physiology, were shown how to give chloroform by rule of thumb. And to say that accidents did not occur was ridiculous and untrue. In Glasgow during a recent year 50 deaths were registered as due to anæsthetics. In 5 months 10 deaths occurred in hospitals alone. In Edinburgh during the past year there have been not less than 6 deaths in public institutions. "Dr. Heron Watson has earned the respect of the whole profession by . . . his brilliant contributions to the surgical art, but a man in his position . . . should make himself more sure of his facts."

Additional evidence in favour of Nicol Jarvie's criticisms came from Professors Glaister and Galt of Glasgow,[9] who stated that, between them, they had done 43 post-mortems on chloroform deaths in Glasgow. So much for the legend of the harmlessness of chloroform on its native soil.

But what on earth possessed Heron Watson to make such a remark in the first place? A blanket-statement such as this, covering a whole country, is obviously, on the face of it, absurd and untrue.

F. W. Hewitt was the first to have some success in a campaign for improvement. By 1907 only 8 out of 27 examining bodies insisted on any evidence of instruction in anæsthetics. After Hewitt's onslaught all bodies demanded this four years later. Hewitt was an outstanding anæsthetist of the old school, who never used spinals or intratracheal methods.

He was the leader of his branch of the profession and was knighted in 1911 for services to Royalty. His controversial style was hard-hitting but completely fair. In 1903 he wrote:[10]

"Whilst it is customary to place at the disposal of hospital patients, so long as they are conscious, the services of the most eminent physicians and surgeons of the day, it is also customary, directly they become unconscious, to hand them over to the care of comparatively uneducated and inexperienced junior officers, who are left to do the best they can for their patients during what may be to the latter the most critical time of their lives. It is difficult to see any reason why the administration of the most powerful agents in the British Pharmacopœia should be placed in the hands of medical men whose qualifications and professional attainments are, as a general rule, inferior to those of other officers."

Every word of this indictment was not only true, but it remained true for a very long time afterwards. Whether it is still true I cannot say. I have been retired from anæsthetics for nearly twenty years.

Perhaps the most cynical and materialistic comment on the matter was made by a surgeon, Sir Alfred Fripp, in 1908. Referring to proposals to improve anæsthesia, he stated that

"it opened up the possibility of having to face a very large social question of whether there was not already more than enough done for that very large class that could afford something but could not afford to pay the full fee for medical and surgical attendance, and who were very prone to get their services for nothing at all."

The Nazi doctors in Belsen and Auschwitz experimented ruthlessly on the lives and health of prisoners who belonged to 'inferior' races. The above opposition to improved anæsthesia because the existing methods were good enough for another 'inferior' race—those who could not afford to pay full fees—does not appear to be very different in principle.

Even to-day traces of the old indifference persist. The usual consent form signed before operation is worded something like this: "I hereby authorise Mr. —— or his proper representative to perform upon my . . . any operation he may deem necessary, and I consent to the administration of an anæsthetic for the purpose of such operation."

Note that permission is given to a named surgeon or his proper representative, but the anæsthetic is left, as far as permission is concerned, to anybody at all, skilled or unskilled, proper or not. And with the usual perversity of things in general, the less skilled and experienced the surgeon, and the more he is in need of every possible help, the less likely he is to get it, as far as the anæsthetic is concerned.

Marshal Joffre, commander of the French Armies in the first World War, said that it took 10,000 to 15,000 lives to train a major-general. It doesn't take as many as that to train an anæsthetist, but it does take a certain number. After all, the anæsthetist takes them one at a time. However incompetent he is, he cannot throw lives away wholesale, as the generals did in the first war, which stands out above all others for the brainless ineptitude with which unprotected human beings were, time after time, month after month, exposed to machine gun fire for years on end, without any tactical or strategical originality of any kind. As a statement about war in general Marshal Joffre's remark sounds reasonable enough. But in this particular war, did it really make much difference whether the general was trained or untrained? Nothing but frontal attacks were ordered, in any case.

I am afraid that surgeons hold a place of unchallenged pre-eminence in a chapter on stupidities. The list is so long that it is difficult to know where to start. Don't blame me. It is not my fault. They *would* pontificate on a subject about which they knew very little. Consequently their opinions are about as valuable as those of an anæsthetist on a purely surgical question.

To take one example at random. A famous German surgeon, in his autobiography,[11] says:

"The operation (for a lung condition) was proceeding normally, when, through a cause we were never able to ascertain, the glowing cautery set light to the ether vapour used as the anæsthetic. The violent explosion that followed was repeated almost immediately as an oxygen cylinder blew up. The patient was killed on the spot, the sister and the assistant were injured, and I lost an eardrum."

This is exactly like saying, "I dropped a lighted match into the petrol tank, when, through a cause we were never able to ascertain, the car caught fire." Comment appears to be unnecessary.

In this connection one may also mention once more Lawson Tait's ether apparatus, in which ether in a glass vessel is supposed to be vapourised by the open flame of a spirit lamp![12]

Deloup[13] used 4% cocaine for spinal anæsthesia in the early days of the method. After 100 cases he concluded that it was as safe or safer than general anæsthesia. His experience of general anæsthesia must have been indeed unfortunate.

This somewhat premature optimism reminds one of Sir James Simpson in his original account of a new anæsthetic (chloroform).[14] "I am enabled to speak most confidently of its superior anæsthetic properties, having now tried it upon upwards of thirty individuals."

Or of H. Tyrrell Gray,[15] who reported 200 cases of spinal stovaine in children, and claimed that there was no risk of pulmonary complications or of dangers due to status lymphaticus. I know of no figures of the incidence of status lymphaticus, but I do not think that anybody ever claimed for it an incidence as frequent as 1 in 200.

M. Reynier[16] used a new chloroform inhaler 125 times and described it as "free from danger." Always remember that chloroform at its worst was never accused of a mortality of more than one in a thousand, or even two thousand.

Professor Thomas Jonnesco[17] claimed for his total spinal anæsthesia, which anæsthetised the whole body, "General spinal anæsthesia is absolutely safe; it has never caused death, nor produced any important complications, early or late . . . is infinitely superior to general anæsthesia . . . there are no contraindications. . . ." All this after just over 400 cases! I don't really think that I would welcome the idea of a mastoid operation under spinal anæsthesia, would you?

Dr. P. M. Chapman,[18] Physician to the Herefordshire General Hospital, was even more modest in his safety requirements. He borrowed Dubois' percentage chloroform apparatus—a large and heavy machine—from a physiological laboratory, and also borrowed the physiologist, Dr. Waller, who actually used the machine while Dr. Chapman watched and took notes. He was "greatly struck by . . . the maintenance of the anæsthesia upon a smooth plane. . . . Throughout there was a quite extraordinary absence of anxiety." The modesty of his demands will be appreciated when it is realised that these pæans of praise are bestowed upon a total experience of five cases. How many desperate emergencies did he expect to meet in that number? As regards his criteria of smooth anæsthesia the severity of these may be judged from his report. Out of five cases two of them moved on incision and one vomited during the operation.

But he persevered with the method and five years later[19] he reported his experience "in many hundreds of cases." It was still favourable, with a little more justification this time. Presumably the tame physiologist had been allowed to return to his laboratory after teaching Dr. Chapman all about anæsthesia in five cases, for there is no further mention of him.

It must have been a great comfort to hundreds of doctors whose patients had died under their hands to listen to Edward Lawrie,[20] of Hyderabad, the great protagonist of chloroform—"It is clear from Dr. Colin Smith's account of the case that the heart was refusing to convey any more chloroform to the brain. . . . If the patient had only been left alone . . . *the stoppage of the heart would have saved his life.*" (My italics.)

Dr. Meggison would have loved to hear this.

Professor A. D. Waller[21] ridiculed the idea of reflex arrest of the heart in light anæsthesia—a thing which was reported every week in the medical press—"as well expect a man to be intoxicated because he has taken too little whisky." But then Professor Waller did not deal with patients. He was incarcerated behind the walls of a laboratory, perhaps studying the effect of cantharides upon the hedgehog.

As Henry K. Beecher said, nearly forty years later,[22] laboratory workers demonstrated the effects of overdosage of chloroform and assumed that this covered everything. But the clinicians knew that this was not so—the physiologists had only covered one third of the problem. They were quite right as far as they went—overdosage could and did occur, much more easily with chloroform than with any other anæsthetic, because it was by far the strongest, but that was not the whole story. They omitted from their calculations both primary cardiac failure and delayed chloroform poisoning.

It is not often that one has the opportunity, a century later, to trace the actual degeneration of a first class brain due to age, as certainly as if one had performed a post-mortem on the body and found arterio-sclerosis. Mr. Thomas Nunneley, F.R.C.S., was born in March, 1809. He was, like many medical men of his age, a specialist in everything. He was an ophthalmic surgeon who did over a thousand cataract oper-ations. He was a general surgeon—surgeon to the Leeds Infirmary from 1864. He had a special leaning towards toxicology. He was also Lecturer in surgery and anatomy at the Medical School. And, like all the other members of the staff at that period, he was also in general practice. His capacity for work must have been tremendous.

A man of this calibre was very receptive to new ideas—up to a point and up to a certain age. It so happened that his working life covered the introduction of the two great advances of surgery during the nineteenth century. But his reception of them was very different. In 1849 he was forty years old, and he began with great enthusiasm to investigate the new science of anæsthesia, with the laudable intention of improving it. He tried many new anæsthetic substances, including ethylene, which he rejected as useless. It must be remembered that oxygen was not easily available in those days—if you wanted it you had to make it, collect it and store it yourself. It was over seventy years later before Arno Luckhardt re-investigated ethylene and put it on the map again. But, by this time, when he needed oxygen all he had to do was to telephone and as many cylinders as he liked would be delivered promptly. This simplified things. Nunneley had better results with chloride of olefiant gas or Dutch oil and with coal gas. He thought the latter was cheap, which it was, effective, which it was—often permanently so—safe, which is doubtful, and manageable, which is very questionable. He published a book on his researches.[23]

So he was a thoroughly progressive man, open-minded and willing to accept, or at least to examine, anything new. But, twenty years later, in 1869, when he was sixty, his attitude had changed altogether. His receptiveness had disappeared completely and he had developed into a die-hard obstructionist. Perhaps it is not to be wondered at considering his manifold activities, which were sufficient to wear out any human being.

Hear what he has to say about the second great advance of surgery—the antiseptic system:[24] "During the last three years, since the 'antiseptic treatment' has been in vogue, I have not allowed one of my patients to be treated with carbolic acid; while my colleagues have very extensively employed it . . . my cases without it are as good as theirs with it."

Lister,[25] very justifiably, treated this argument as it deserved to be treated: "That he should dogmatically oppose a treatment which he so little understands, and which by his own admission he has never tried, is a matter of small moment—" and dismissed the matter.

Stupidity shows itself in many ways. The men who claim perfect safety for their methods after a mere handful of cases, and the men who push a red-hot cautery into an ether-filled mouth and wonder why the patient belches fire and flames, are by no means unique in their folly.

Albert H. Miller, of Providence, R.I.,[26] an anæsthetist, uncovers another instance of imbecility. Referring to a period just before the first World War he says:

"Soon more than a thousand gas oxygen machines had been sold in this country. As there were fewer than a hundred professional anæsthetists at the time, most of these machines must have been acquired by surgeons, clinics and hospitals. . . . Hospital authorities met complaints of the quality of anæsthesia by the purchase of more expensive and more complicated gas machines, not recognising the evident fact that safety in anæsthesia abides not in apparatus but in those who use it."

This particular form of half-wittedness has been dealt with so efficiently and so adequately by Sir Robert Macintosh[27] that I do not think I can, or need, add anything to his comments:

"In the immediate post-war years distinguished foreign surgeons visiting clinics in England and the North American continent often commented on the fact that the uniform smoothness of the anæsthesia contrasted with the bouts of turbulence which prevailed from time to time in their own operating theatres. The visitor tended to attribute the credit for this to the apparatus in use, and not to the man behind it. It followed naturally that he should order one of these chromium plated monsters for himself; and he was surprised, and indeed, disgruntled, when it failed to deliver the goods in his own clinic. . . . I have seen one such machine in a corner of an operating theatre, where it had remained for months after dispatching an unfortunate victim who might have survived the insult of open ether. How much better it would have been if that hospital had bought simpler apparatus and spent the balance of the money on training someone to use it properly."

Another group of fatuities is due to lack of chemical or physiological knowledge. George Bodington[28] stated that bad anæsthetic results were not due to the anæsthetic itself but to the lack of oxygen which accompanied it. "The chloroform gas occupies all the air passages to the exclusion of the atmosphere, and consequently oxygen, and the patient is at once in danger of being asphyxiated." How unfortunate that he should have chosen chloroform to illustrate his argument. From its very strength and the small amount of it required it could not possibly act in this way. It was before the era of Vernon Harcourt's inhaler, which limited the strength of the vapour to 2%, but there was no real excuse for Mr. Bodington's ignorance. Long before his time John Snow had worked out the strength of chloroform vapour needed for anæsthesia and had shown that the absolute maximum for safety was 5%. This amount could only reduce the oxygen content of the inspired air by about one per cent.

Moreover Mr. Bodington continues, stepping cheerfully from the frying pan of bad physics into the fire of worse chemistry: "I do not understand the more perfect safety of the nitrous oxide gas, except that it conveys more free oxygen into the system when inspired." He ignored the fact that the oxygen in nitrous oxide is not free but combined, so that it is not available to the body at body temperatures.

Thomas W. Evans,[29] the American dentist from Paris, who gave demonstrations in London and was thereby responsible for the re-birth of nitrous oxide in England after it had been neglected and forgotten for twenty years, stated that nitrous oxide contains a larger proportion of oxygen than exists in atmospheric air, and it therefore supports combustion. It does, of course, at temperatures high enough to dissociate it, but not at body temperature, when the oxygen content of it is firmly combined and quite useless to the body metabolism.

A. Ernest Sansom[30] replied to this in the next week's issue by stating that nitric acid contains still more oxygen than either of the two gases mentioned; therefore it should be better and safer than both! Dr. Sansom had done quite a lot of work on chloroform a few years before and had written a very good book on it.[31] He did not like nitrous oxide at all.

Dr. Kidd[32] referred to chloroform as a test for epilepsy, and to experiments made in France on this subject. If a patient feigned to be the subject of epilepsy, he said, the administration of chloroform did not induce a seizure; whilst the contrary was the case when the patient was really epileptic. John Snow very emphatically and rightly disagreed, on the very valid ground that the facts were not correct. "It was no test, and was a most unjustifiable proceeding. He had often given chloroform to persons subject to epilepsy, and they had become quietly insensible and slept as did other patients."

A distinguished physiologist, Schaefer,[33] fell into the same sort of trap. He knew that chloroform caused a steady fall in blood pressure; he also knew that supra-renal extract—this was before adrenalin itself was isolated—raised the blood pressure most efficiently. He therefore suggested supra-renal extract as an antidote to chloroform. He had the excuse that this was years before Goodman Levy demonstrated the dangerous synergism of these two drugs and their liability to cause fatal ventricular fibrillation.

Attempts at prophecy also led to stupid statements on occasion. Mr. Erichsen, one of the foremost surgeons of the day, stated in 1873[34] that the knife could not always have fresh fields to conquer—that the limit had nearly, if not quite, been reached. "If we reflect on the great achievements of modern operative surgery, very little remains for the boldest to devise, or for the most dexterous to perform."

One of his house surgeons, later Sir St. Clair Thomson, recalled this speech 65 years later—in 1938.[35] Erichsen's recorded amputation mortality was 25%, which he considered a very satisfactory result. Also, according to Thomson, he predicted that "the abdomen, the chest and the brain would be for ever shut from the intrusion of the wise and humane surgeon."

Could Erichsen have chosen a worse moment for his rash prophecies? Surgeons were not, as he thought, at the end of surgery, but at its very beginning, thanks to Lister, who was even then experimenting and struggling to get his revolutionary ideas accepted.

Still, he may be forgiven, for over forty years later, when aseptic surgery had conquered the world and extended the bounds of surgery into all the territories which Erichsen had thought to be for ever untouchable, there were still loopholes in aseptic technique.

F. St. J. Steadman,[36] a dental surgeon, pointed out some of them. He saw nine consecutive cases in a London Hospital die after major operation on the tongue and mouth, due to sepsis caused by pyorrhœa. Then in a further five cases he extracted all teeth and stumps a week or ten days before operation. All these cases recovered. "It is difficult to understand the attitude of the surgeon who takes infinite precautions to sterilise the area of operation before making a skin incision and who yet will perform an extensive operation in the mouth actually in the presence of pus."

Mistakes made by a surgeon can usually be rectified by a more skilful surgeon at a later date—they are not very often fatal. An anæsthetist's mistakes, on the other hand, tend to be permanent and final, because they are fatal. Not always, but frequently. This being so, it is strange that so many attempts have been made either to dispense with his services altogether or to dispense with or discourage his adequate training. It has always been the same throughout the first century of anæsthesia, and almost all over the world.

Jonnesco,[37] in addition to his ridiculous claim for complete safety for his very high spinal anæsthesia after a very small experience of the method, made an even more absurd claim in its favour—"it does away with the attendance of a person often inexperienced and never responsible." It did not occur to him for a moment that if his anæsthetists were of this calibre, the fault was entirely his own for allowing it.

Thomas Annandale,[38] Professor of Clinical Surgery, Edinburgh, had a rather similar outlook. If one may so describe it, it was in his case an attitude of very honest stupidity, because he was prepared to stake his own life on this belief. "Chloroform holds the field as the best general anæsthetic in connexion with surgical procedures"; he said,

"and although I have met with a few fatal results from its administration I have most thorough confidence in its safety if carefully used and its effects diligently watched. Perhaps the best test of my confidence is the fact that . . . I required to take an anæsthetic on several occasions . . . the anæsthetic I took was chloroform; and it was administered according to the open method by one of my assistants and not by a special anæsthetist."

I respect the honesty of his opinions more than I respect the intellect which arrived at them.

The Worcester General Infirmary decided to sack its anæsthetist in 1900. *The Lancet* commented that it was a retrograde step.[39]

Another attempt to abolish the anæsthetist was made in 1939.[40] A surgeon designed a sort of 'draw-over' ether apparatus which could be used single handed as it worked automatically. The same author, three years later,[41] in an article on tonsillectomy, admitted that a specialist anæsthetist gave much better results. "Many years ago, when changing house surgeons gave the anæsthetics, we had one or two fatalities, but for five years, since this anæsthetist has been doing this work we have had none."

No figures are given, except for the airy reference to "one or two fatalities," so the testimonial is not of much scientific value.

Examples of confused thinking are common. J. H. Marsh[42] explains that the earliest effect of an overdose of chloroform is arterio-capillary contraction, which is a sort of stopcock action in order to prevent the blood, dangerously loaded with chloroform, from reaching the tissues. Amyl nitrite is valuable in treatment by relaxing the contraction, states the author, and thereby, if his theory is true, liberating a dangerous dose of chloroform to the tissues.

Sir William Mitchell Banks, the Liverpool surgeon,[43] who had been house surgeon to Syme and had no doubt imbibed his doctrine of plenty of air and plenty of chloroform, pointed out the danger of taking a long time to put the patient under with small does of chloroform, for by the time anæsthesia was produced the patient had inhaled a large quantity and had gone under very deeply! If a too cautious student doled out the chloroform drop by drop so slowly that at the end of thirty minutes the patient was not under, what difference would this amount of wasted anæsthetic make if someone then came along and chloroformed the patient to the third stage in six minutes?

Sir Lauder Brunton, echoing Lawrie, said that ether could not be used in very hot climates. It would have been better if they had taken John Hunter's advice, "Don't think. Try it." J. E. Squire[44] tried it in 1885. He gave ether in Suakim for all operations in the Suakim Field Force. He only used chloroform once. The temperature was over 100° and sometimes over 120° in the shade. He found that larger quantities were used, but there was no difficulty.

My own experience of open ether under these conditions is confined to one emergency case in Ceylon in August, and to 61 cases in Greece during the four hot months (June to September). Most of the patients were managed under evipan or pentothal and/or gas and oxygen, so ether was not often used, but sufficiently often to prove that chloroform is not necessary for climatic reasons alone. I noticed no difficulty with ether.

But are anæsthetists immune from silly sayings and stupid doings? By no means, although I have not been able to find examples quite so easily as amongst non-anæsthetists, who seem particularly liable to make dogmatic statements on a subject they know little about.

Richard Gill,[45] anæsthetist to St. Bartholomew's Hospital from 1893-1916, was on doubtful ground when he said that "chloroform acted upon the cerebral centres solely by reason of its chemical action on the blood. When chloroform was absorbed by the blood it was oxidised by the nascent oxygen in the blood, and this loss of oxygen . . . caused chloroform narcosis." Dudley Buxton objected to this, for the very good reason that chloroform narcosis still occurs just as easily if oxygen was given along with the chloroform.

John Snow himself was guilty of one or two rather outrageous statements, although most of his work was very sound and most of his writings sane and sensible to the last degree. He said, in the very early days, that he had never seen any operation under . . . ether or chloroform where stimulants seemed required. . . . He had never given drink to patients when insensible; but if it were thought necessary, there would be no danger in doing so, as a small quantity of liquid would run down the œsophagus, even if the patient could not swallow it. The hypodermic syringe was not yet born when he said this.[46]

Perhaps he was right, at the time he wrote. In 1848 there was no such thing as deep anæsthesia, and it is just possible that he could have got away with it. After all, for many years he gave chloroform to patients for mouth operations and kept the airway free from blood, in the absence of any other protection, by tilting the head forward at intervals (in the sitting position) and partly by such light anæsthesia that the cough reflex was not abolished. No doubt many of these patients swallowed a good deal of blood.

His habit of using chloroform in the upright position was one of the few things in his practice to which exception might be taken—but he never had a fatality from it. At least he could and did tackle these difficult cases, unlike Syme, who stuck with incredible stubbornness to his dogma that anybody could give chloroform. If they couldn't, that is if it was a difficult case, such as a removal of the upper jaw, the answer was, not to get an expert to do the job, but to operate without any anæsthetic at all. Syme continued this brutal and unnecessary practice for years after Snow had successfully tackled these cases.

Another early statement made by Snow is open to doubt. After eight years' experience he said that death from mental emotion could not happen with chloroform[47] "as the patient neither feels nor thinks when fully under the influence of chloroform." The trouble was that patients died before they were fully under. But Snow was lucky enough never to meet with one of these tragic cases.

About 1932 chloroform capsules, containing 20 minims, were introduced—not by an anæsthetist—as a means whereby midwives could satisfy the increasing demand for analgesia in labour. It has always seemed to me that to issue to nurses without supervision the one drug which had been given up by expert anæsthetists all over the world as dangerous, was not a very intelligent thing to do.

Examples of stupidity could be multiplied without end.

One of the most astounding examples of resistance to new ideas occurred just before Lord Nuffield founded the first Professorship of Anæsthesia in this country.[48] Lord Nuffield gave £2,000,000 to Oxford University, in order, among other things, to endow medical professorships, including a chair of anæsthetics.[49] The inclusion of anæsthetics was directly due to Nuffield's enlightened insistence. He had had personal experience of anæsthetics on several occasions, both skilfully and unskilfully administered, and the difference must have impressed him considerably.

Although doubt was expressed whether anæsthetics was really a suitable subject for a chair, Nuffield persisted in his view that it would benefit from a professor who could devote himself whole-heartedly to its advancement through teaching and research. He remembers walking up and down with Sir Farquhar Buzzard, the Regius Professor of Medicine, arguing, and finally making it clear that he felt so strongly about it that his backing of the whole scheme would otherwise be in doubt. In this way Oxford got the first chair in anæsthetics in the British Commonwealth.

This enlightened and strong-minded action by a layman forced this great advance into being against the opposition of one who should, above all others, have been receptive of new ideas—especially when some one else was prepared to pay for them.

I notice, *en passant*, that seven years before[50] an address was published entitled, *Arrogance and ignorance in medicine*, by Sir Farquhar Buzzard, Bart., Consulting Physician to St. Thomas's Hospital and Regius Professor of Medicine in the University of Oxford.

Tom Bird,[51] Instructor in the use of anæsthetics to Guy's Hospital, commenting on Flux's open gas apparatus, stated that his own gas apparatus, designed twenty years before, could be used in the same way. But the open method was very extravagant, so he had never published it. "I do not think the fees admit such a waste of gas." He goes on to say that Clover once told him that the use of dichloride of ethidene once cost him thirty shillings out of a two guinea fee ($7.20 out of 10 dollars).

It should be self-evident that it is a dangerous absurdity if an anæsthetist has to consider pennies when dealing with human lives. At the best, from an idealistic point of view, this should never happen to anybody, anywhere. From a more material view-point, and considering private patients only, most of them were paying very large fees for extra special attention, and in fact were getting the cheapest possible service, as far as the anæsthetic was concerned.

An experience of my own is very much to the point here. When I was an anæsthetist I had to be in general practice as well. I possessed two gas oxygen machines, which at that time cost me 25/- an hour to use, counting the cost of gases consumed, together with maintenance, transport and depreciation. These could be used only in my anæsthetic practice. For general practice they were out of the question, partly because of their size and weight, but largely because of their high running cost.

One night I was called in—as a G.P.—to give an anæsthetic for a confinement. This meant two or three hours off my night's sleep for a fee of 21/-. Gas and oxygen would have cost more than the fee. So I gave chloroform for a forceps delivery. That patient died a few days later from delayed chloroform poisoning—the only one I have ever seen, I am glad to say.

To crown the absurdity and tragedy of the whole thing, a consultant obstetrician was called in to see the patient, in spite of the fact that all treatment was known to be useless, and he was paid, for doing nothing at a time convenient to himself, exactly five times the fee I got for giving the anæsthetic in the middle of the night!

This was one of the reasons why I got out of anæsthesia altogether. I thought it was about time, when totally unnecessary deaths were caused by cheese-paring financial considerations.

Having quoted many stupidities and absurdities committed by others —with references to substantiate them—I thought, in all fairness, that I should add one of my own, lest it be thought that I am claiming to be infallible.

REFERENCES

[1] *Lancet* (1858), Sept. 4. 261.

[2] *Lancet* (1858), Oct. 30. 457.

[3] *Lancet* (1854), Nov. 11. 404.

[4] *Lancet* (1858), Sept. 18. 314.

[5] *Lancet* (1858), Oct. 9. 389.

[6] *Lancet* (1882), Dec. 23. 1070.

[7] *Lancet* (1889), Sept. 14. 564.

[8] *Lancet* (1902), Jan. 11. 122.

[9] *Lancet* (1903), April 25. 1183.

[10] *Lancet* (1903), Dec. 12. 1683.

[11] Ferdinand Sauerbruch. *A Surgeon's Life.*

[12] *Lancet* (1876), May 13. 721.

[13] *Med. Annu.* (1906). 461.

[14] Paper read before the Edinburgh Medico-chirurgical Society. (1847), Nov. 10.

[15] *Lancet* (1909), Oct. 2. 991.

[16] *Lancet* (1905), Feb. 25. 533.

[17] *Brit. med. J.* (1909), Nov. 13. 1399.

[18] *Lancet* (1904), Jan. 16. 153.

[19] *Lancet* (1909), Jan. 9. 91.

[20] *Lancet* (1892), July 9. 115.

[21] *Lancet* (1904), Oct. 1. 978.

[22] *Anæsthesiology* (1941). Vol. 2. 447.

[23] *On Anæsthesia and anæsthetic substances.*

[24] *Brit. med. J.* (1869), Aug. 7. 156.

[25] *Med. Tms. Gaz.* (1869), Aug. 28. 265.

[26] *Anæsthesiology* (1941). Vol. 2. 404.

[27] *Brit. med. J.* (1955), Oct. 29. 1054.

[28] *Lancet* (1873), Jan. 4. 32.

[29] *Brit. med. J.* (1868), May 2. 436.

[30] *Brit. med. J.* (1868), May 9. 462.

[31] *Chloroform: its action and administration* (1865). 187 pages. London. John Churchill.

[32] *Lancet* (1856), Nov. 29. 599.

[33] *Lancet* (1899), Dec. 30. 1832.

[34] *Lancet* (1873), Oct. 4. Introductory address. University College Hospital.

[35] *Lancet* (1938), Oct. 15. 911.

[36] *Lancet* (1914), Jan. 3. 74.

[37] *Brit. med. J.* (1909), Nov. 13. 1399.

[38] *Lancet* (1898), July 30. 249.

[39] *Lancet* (1900), Dec. 22. 1828.

[40] *Brit. med. J.* (1939), May 27. 1110.

[41] *Brit. med. J.* (1942), Oct. 31. 512.

[42] *Lancet* (1895), Dec. 7. 1481.

[43] *Lancet* (1901), May 11. 1339.

[44] *Lancet* (1890), Feb. 22, 434; and 1913, May 17, 1415.

[45] *Lancet* (1908), Nov. 14. 1445.

[46] *Lancet* (1848). I. 312.

[47] *Lancet* (1855), Oct. 20. 361.

[48] P. W. S. Andrews and Elizabeth Brunner. *The Life of Lord Nuffield.* 289 pages. Basil Blackwell.

[49] *Lancet* (1936), Oct.

[50] *Lancet* (1929), Oct. 5. 694.

[51] *Lancet* (1898), Oct. 15. 1021, or Oct. 8. 933.

CHAPTER 7

THE SEVEN FOUNDATION STONES;
IN ORDER OF MERIT

"Let us now praise famous men. . . . "
—ECCLESIASTICUS 44. 1.

T
HE seven pioneers of anæsthesia, are, of course, Davy, Hickman, Long and Wells, followed by the inseparable enemies Morton and Jackson, and lastly Simpson. That is their chronological order, with dates ranging from 1799 to 1847. Two country general practitioners, two dentists, two chemists and an obstetrician. Four Americans and three British. Such were the men who made painless surgery possible. Thousands of words have been written about them and their contributions to the discovery. No doubt thousands more will be added to the controversy. I propose to add a few myself.

To arrange them in order of merit is not easy. Whatever facts are brought forward, whatever arguments are used, the question will always remain highly debatable. My own feeling is that they should be ranked thus, in descending order of importance; first Hickman, then Wells, Morton, Davy, Long, Simpson, and, a long way last, Jackson. This ranking takes into account not only their originality but the amount of work they did, their attempts to publicise their work, the amount of luck they had, and lastly their courage.

For no amount of originality is of use to the world if the world never hears about it, or if the idea dies with its inventor. Again, no amount of work for an ideal is of any avail if the idealist is dogged persistently by bad luck. It is not claimed that this, or any other, assessment is final or infallible. All that can be said is that a reasoned case can be made out for it.

Henry Hill Hickman (1800-1830) was born at Lady Halton, a charming seventeenth century farmhouse near the village of Bromfield, which is about two miles from Ludlow in Shropshire. He died at Tenbury Wells, where he was in practice at 18 Teme Street, and was buried in Bromfield churchyard. His tombstone, much weathered, has been transferred to the shelter of the church porch and a tablet has been put up to his memory in the church itself.

He above all others had the idea of anæsthesia most deeply and spontaneously engrained in him, and hence he had the most originality of mind. It must be remembered that in his time the idea was not floating about in the air, so to speak, as it was in the eighteen forties. It simply just did not exist at all, except in his imagination. He died a short ten years too early for that. All the other candidates (except Davy) lived at a time when medical students' ether frolics and itinerant showmen like Colton were accidentally and quite unwittingly paving the way for something deeper, for something really important, for a revolution of practical utility. And so for pure originality of thought Hickman stands supreme. He alone conceived the idea without external stimulus of any kind.

His predecessor Davy happened, it is true, to discover the narcotic action of nitrous oxide accidentally during his chemical researches into the preparation and nature of the gas—a nice example of serendipity. But he merely noted the fact briefly and passed on to something else. The thought made no real impression on his mind.

Great as the merits of Wells and Morton were they had only to seize upon and develop an idea which was already beginning to crystallise. Hickman did not even have this advantage. If one excludes mediæval and mythical fables about mandragora and the *spongia somnifera*, which have been stressed in the history books to an extent out of all proportion to their importance, which was nil, the only previous reference of any value at all in world literature was one solitary sentence in Davy's book.

It is certain that Hickman had never heard of this, or there would have been more about nitrous oxide in his notebooks. He would surely have abandoned his unsatisfactory carbon dioxide in favour of something more promising, if he had known about it or even suspected it.

It was not possible to buy the gas at that time or for half a century afterwards, but it was not difficult to make, and an enthusiast like Hickman could have made it and used it easily enough, as Davy had done before him and as thousands of dentists did forty years later, until the introduction of iron cylinders about 1870 made it an article of commerce.

Not only did Hickman spend much time experimenting with his chosen gas, but he tried hard to bring the idea to public notice. As a young and obscure general practitioner and probably not a very successful one, for he practised in three different places in his working life of ten years, he took the trouble and faced the expense of having his work printed as a booklet in 1824, so as to bring it to the notice of Mr. T. A.

Knight, who was the local squire of Downton Castle and one of the Presidents of the Royal Society. What a pity Knight did not take more interest in it. He could so easily have had a word with Davy, his co-Fellow, who lived until 1829. Davy would certainly have suggested nitrous oxide.

When this seed fell upon stony ground Hickman petitioned Charles X of France, in 1828. The King, more impressed or more intelligent than Mr. Knight, brought the idea to the notice of French scientists. But all to no purpose. They were not interested, with the exception of Baron Larrey, who had some experience of natural anæsthesia due to extreme cold during Napoleon's disastrous retreat from Russia.

What more could poor Hickman do? He was a busy man, who had to earn his living in poorly paid work; he was tied hand and foot to his practice. Moreover he died at the age of thirty. He had not much time at his disposal.

The amount of work he did was large, considering his short life and his commitments as a general practitioner. Courage did not enter into his work at all, as there is no evidence that he experimented on himself, nor did he experiment on other human beings. He never got as far as that, for he was the victim of very bad luck. He chose carbon dioxide as his agent. Whilst it gave him results sufficiently good to keep his interest alive, it was really a most unfortunate choice—a very poor, uncontrollable and dangerous gas to use.

But he did enough, considering all these things, to put him right at the top of the list, in spite of the fact that his work did not lead directly to any practical results. After all success alone is not always the ultimate criterion. Few people would argue that Wellington was a better general than Napoleon because he beat the Emperor at Waterloo. And Robert E. Lee ranks very high among the great Captains even though his career ended in defeat and surrender.

Horace Wells was born in 1815 and died by his own hand on January 24th, 1848, at the age of 33. He was a dentist in Hartford, Connecticut. He gets almost full marks for the originality of his idea, but not quite, say seven out of ten. He lacked the spontaneous genius of Hickman. He did not think of anæsthesia at all until he had seen Colton's public exhibition of the effect of inhaling nitrous oxide, which visited Hartford on December 10th, 1844. But, given this stimulus and the sight of a man partly under the influence of gas failing to notice an injury, he saw the possibilities of it at once, as no one else had done. So much so that he arranged for a personal trial of it for the very next day. On that eventful

Wednesday Colton gave him the gas for the removal of a tooth, watched by Mr. Cooley, the man who had unconsciously injured his leg on the previous evening.

Colton, on the other hand, had never appreciated the potential value of his gas at all. He had looked upon it merely as a fairground sideshow and as a living for himself as a showman, and nothing more. All he had proved, all he had learnt, was that nitrous oxide could be safely inhaled and that it was an intoxicant of sorts. This was much less than Davy knew about it forty-five years before. The idea of making practical use of his inhalations, the idea of anæsthesia itself, had obviously never entered his head, in spite of the fact that he had lived so long on the very borderline of the new discovery. If he had thought of it he would assuredly have tried it, with the help of some doctor or dentist, as he in fact tried it with, and on the person of, Horace Wells.

To do him justice as an honest man, and he was honest, never at any time did he claim any merit as a pioneer. He was astute enough to put his gas to practical use during the years which followed, as soon as the idea had been pointed out to him by a man with a more original mind, for he formed the Colton Dental Association, with branches in seven of the largest cities of the United States. This institution specialised in painless dentistry under nitrous oxide, and Colton no doubt did very well out of it. But beyond this he claimed nothing. Though a minor character in the drama, and not one of the real pioneers, he comes out of it with an unblemished reputation. He was not grasping or unscrupulous, which is more than can be said for some of the others.

As regards the amount of work put into the discovery Wells was somewhat careless and over-confident. After his personal experience of anæsthesia and a very small amount of practice in administering it to patients—about fifteen cases—he went off at half-cock and gave his disastrous public demonstration at the Massachusetts General Hospital in January, 1845.

This failure, or partial failure, wrecked his chances for ever and led ultimately to his tragic suicide. If only he had had a little patience and gained more knowledge and more experience before trying to convert the world to the agony of a new idea! With the wisdom which comes so easily after the event, and with the accumulated experience of over a hundred years to help us it is simple enough to recognise the difficulties which he failed to foresee. Nitrous oxide is the weakest of all anæsthetics and by far the most difficult to control, partly because of its gaseous state and partly because of its lack of power. It is so often used today preceded

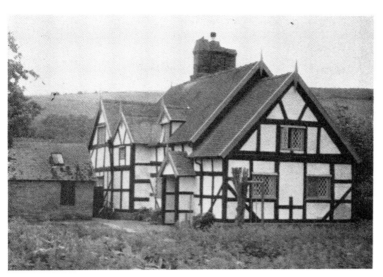

PLATE XXV.—Henry Hill Hickman's birthplace. Lady Halton, a farmhouse near Bromfield, Ludlow; built in 1687.

Photograph by the author.

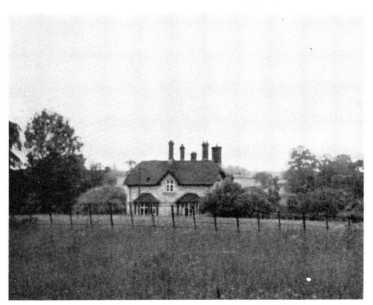

PLATE XXVI.—Downton Castle, Herefordshire, near Bromfield. The residence of Mr. T. A. Knight, the local squire, to whom Hickman addressed his experiments in vain.

Photograph taken by the author.

facing page 120

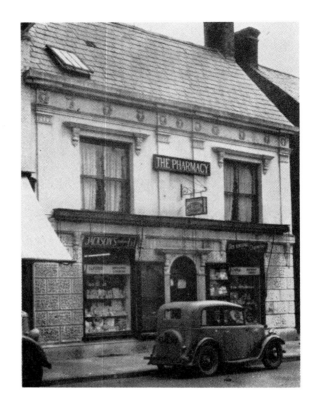

PLATE XXVII

Hickman started practice in Ludlow in 1820.
In 1824 he removed to Shifnal. Later he moved
to this house, 18 Teme Street, Tenbury Wells.
He died here at the age of 30.

Photograph taken by the author

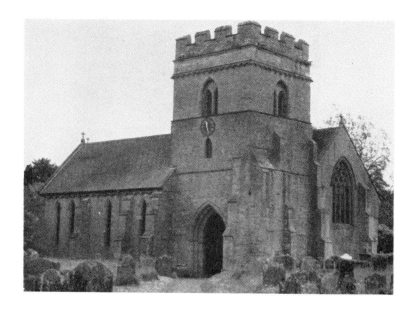

PLATE XXVIII

Hickman was buried in the churchyard of the Church of
St. Mary the Virgin, at Bromfield. *Photograph taken by the
author, by permission of the Rev. Peter Nourse.*

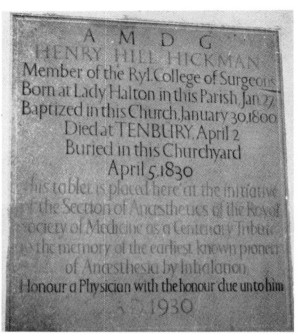

PLATE XXIX.—This memorial tablet is in the church itself. *Photograph taken by the author.*

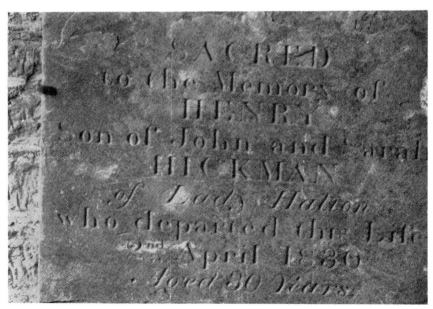

PLATE XXX.—The gravestone of Henry Hill Hickman. It has been weathered considerably, but is now in the porch of Bromfield Church in a protected position. The 30 in the bottom line looks very like 80 except with a magnifying glass. *Photograph taken by the author.*

by and mixed with so many other drugs as adjuvants that it is possible to forget that, even with the best modern apparatus it is not always easy to get a tranquil gas anæsthesia with gas *alone* in an unpremedicated patient. Even the expert runs into trouble occasionally, or has to add some more powerful drug. And Wells was by no means an expert, but a mere novice at the time. And he had nothing in reserve to add to his gas in case of need.

Moreover his apparatus was laughably crude and impossibly primitive. It consisted of a simple animal bladder full of gas with a wooden tube tied into it. This tube the patient had to hold in his mouth, while his nose was compressed by a clip or by the finger and thumb of an assistant. Uncomfortable and psychologically upsetting, to say the least of it. Besides, no one knew how much air leaked round the mouthpiece or how much rebreathing took place. Probably a good deal of both, in varying proportions, never twice the same.

All anæsthetists know in their heart of hearts that the man behind the machine is far more important than the machine itself. (Although, judging by the vast number of anæsthetic apparatuses designed by and constructed by anæsthetists it would appear that this knowledge is frequently forgotten.) But it is also true that, the less power the anæsthetic possesses the more important it is that the machine should be efficient in order to extract from its weakness the utmost results which the drug is capable of giving. Only with the stronger agents is it possible to improvise an apparatus out of almost anything at hand and get fairly good results.

Premedication was unheard of; experience was very limited; nothing was known about which type of patient was likely to be resistant and which were the easy ones. Add to this the natural tension and excitement of a public demonstration, when everything is likely to go wrong, and the result was inevitable. Moreover it was not an ordinary demonstration, but something revolutionary, something incredible, something utterly unheard of, performed before an audience of unbelievers, to whom the thought of painless surgery was merely a bad joke or the dream of a madman. But Wells was not mad—not yet.

Wells had shot his bolt when his demonstration failed to convince the diehards. He continued to believe in his discovery, with good reason. He knew that it worked, he knew it was practical. But after his public humiliation he had not the heart to go on. He was not a strong enough character to fight against adversary or to combat unbelief.

His luck was bad, in that he used a weak and technically difficult anæsthetic, and used it prematurely. Courage he had, at any rate at the beginning, for he was the first human being to have a tooth extracted under gas. But he had not the enduring type of courage—or is it merely thickness of skin?—which Simpson showed when he fought the adversaries of chloroform tooth and nail. One cannot imagine the massive Simpson being depressed or committing suicide because of a bad anæsthesia.

But nothing can rob Wells of the honour of being the first person to use anæsthesia effectively, who at the same time tried to introduce his discovery to the world. The fact that he failed hardly matters.

W. T. G. Morton (1819-1868) does not take a high place for originality, but for other reasons. He got the idea of anæsthesia itself from Wells, with whom he had been in partnership. When Wells failed to arouse interest or even belief in anæsthesia and dropped out of the picture, it was merely a question of looking for a more efficient substitute. Ether was suggested to Morton, either by the ether parties of the medical students, which were now common knowledge, or by Jackson the chemist. If Jackson did make this suggestion it was about all he did do, in spite of his later bombastic and extravagant claims.

Morton did a little work on animals and on himself, but not a great deal. He knew very little about ether when he anæsthetised his first patient, Eben Frost, for the removal of a tooth, on 30th September, 1846. A fortnight later, on 16th October, he demonstrated his new method at the Massachusetts General Hospital. Rashness and over-confidence? Yes, but as it turned out, not so rash as Wells, for three reasons. One was accidental and due to no merit of his own, in that ether happened to be a more powerful and more manageable agent than nitrous oxide, much more likely to be successful, and much less likely to be affected by primitive or badly designed apparatus. The second reason was, and this is not generally known and not mentioned in any of the histories, that Morton had in fact had a certain amount of practical experience before he gave his famous public demonstration. Dr. W. J. Morton, of New York, said in the *Journal of the American Medical Association* (1911), June 3, 1677: "It is not generally known that previous to the first use of ether at the Massachusetts General Hospital (in 1846) my father, Dr. Morton, had employed this for thirty-seven private operations done by Dr. Henry J. Bigelow, and that, before beginning the administration of ether, he was accustomed to give large doses (40 minims) of laudanum. So it appears that it was Dr. Bigelow who was Morton's first sponsor and not Dr. Warren, as is usually stated and usually believed. It was Warren, of course, who operated on Ether Day, in public.

Perhaps this is why it was left to Dr. Bigelow to write the first descriptive paper about the new process and to send the news to the Old World. It is certainly the first mention of premedication in anæsthesia. This little known fact also explains something which has puzzled me for some time.

Morton's first public demonstration of anæsthesia, on Gilbert Abbott, was not completely successful. The patient did feel something of the skin incision—as though his neck had been scratched with a hoe. Why, then, was not Morton hissed out of the theatre as an impostor in the same way as Wells had been only two years before in the very same place? Remember that audience of cynics and unbelievers—as well they might be. They were being asked to believe the unbelievable, to credit the impossible. Moreover the same trick had been tried on them before. Is it any wonder that they took some convincing?

I think that the answer must lie with Henry J. Bigelow. He must have convinced Warren and the audience that Morton's anæsthesia, even if not perfect, was not a fraud—that he had seen it successful himself in a whole series of cases.

The third reason why Morton was not so rash as Wells was that he was a tougher character, more pushful and less sensitive, and much less easily discouraged. Whatever we may think of his attempt to keep ether a secret under the name of Letheon, and of his patenting it with the idea of drawing world-wide royalties, he fought for his ideas and he fought for his priority. His long continued squabbles with Jackson were not very elevating and not very professional, but at least they led to widespread publicity, even if the attitude of selfishness they introduced lessened the lustre of his achievements to some extent. Rarely has the news of a discovery spread with such speed. It was in use in England and Scotland exactly sixty-four days after the first demonstration in Boston, Mass. Remember that there were no rapid communications and no rapid transport at that time. The Atlantic cable was not laid until nearly twelve years later. Mail boats had steam engines, but they were of low power, and the ships still relied to a large extent on sails, with the result that letters took a fortnight to cross from the States to England.

But even the equable, business-like Morton rushed things a bit, apart from his daring in demonstrating something about which he knew very little. The new inhaler, which was being made for him by Mr. Joseph M. Wightman at the last moment, was barely ready in time, and Morton was in fact late for his historic demonstration. But he was in no way disconcerted. In spite of the rush and hurry of his arrival, in spite of his critical and disbelieving audience, he carried out his first public anæsthesia coolly and sufficiently successfully. This was largely due to the more powerful and more easily handled drug which he used, but was also partly due to his more phlegmatic temperament. His choice of ether was frankly due to luck, of which he had his full share. Anyway, it was about time somebody had some luck in this anæsthesia business.

Morton showed some courage in trying ether on himself, although by this time it was fairly well known to be reasonably safe. There had been no recorded disaster at the ether parties. He showed more courage in his cool demeanour during the ordeal of his first demonstration. Possibly he stressed the commercial aspect of his invention unduly, but he was a poor man, and at that date dentistry had not really reached the status of a profession. It was more a trade or handicraft, learnt like other trades by apprenticeship, with very little in the way of academic knowledge or scientific background. Besides, Morton soon made ample amends for his early unethical conduct. See his original letter about a simple sponge inhaler.

To Morton belongs the undoubted credit of introducing successful anæsthesia with sufficient publicity to ensure that it immediately achieved world-wide acceptance. No longer was there any danger of a great idea being stillborn or dying in infancy. It had already done both of these things.

Sir Humphry Davy (1778-1829) published his book on nitrous oxide in 1800. He stated that his experiments on the gas took him ten months, and the actual writing of the book another three months. So he stands far ahead of all the others as regards the amount of work done on the subject. But he was a chemist, not a doctor or a dentist, and most of his investigations were purely chemical or physical. He did inhale the gas himself on many occasions, after he had tried it on animals of various kinds, including birds, insects and fishes. In this he showed considerable courage, for the gas was reputed to be a deadly poison. In his book* he quotes Samuel Latham Mitchill, who had no doubt whatever about its lethal action and toxic effects.

"If a full inspiration of gaseous oxide be made, there will be a sudden extinction of life; and this accordingly accounts for the fact . . . of many persons falling down dead suddenly, when struck with the contagion of the plague."

*Researches, chemical and philosophical, chiefly concerning nitrous oxide (1800). Republished in his collected works, 1839.

Davy found, however, by experiments on his own person, that not only did he not fall down dead on inhaling it, but also that he did not suffer from the plague.

He also quoted, in addition to his own experiences, descriptions of the effects of nitrous oxide inhalation by eighteen other people, many of whom were—and still are—very well known. S. T. Coleridge and Robert Southey, the poets, Josiah Wedgewood the potter, Robert Kinglake the author of *Eothen,* and Peter Roget of the famous and still used *Thesaurus,* were all brave enough to inhale the supposedly deadly gas and disprove Mr. Mitchill's gloomy and unreliable 'facts'.

He also discovered its analgesic properties, by inhaling it on one occasion when he had toothache, and made his famous suggestion that it could be used for surgical operations "in which no great effusion of blood takes place." Why he made this curious stipulation is not clear. All he knew about its physiological effects was that it would relieve pain. He had done no blood pressure experiments and he was not a physiologist or a practising surgeon.

Having made the suggestion he dropped the matter and took no further steps to follow it up. From one point of view, why should he? It is not fair to expect it from a pure chemist. What is surprising is that his suggestion was completely ignored by the very people whom it should have interested most; that surgeons should have continued, for nearly fifty years longer, to operate upon screaming, struggling patients in full consciousness. Surely a lasting testimonial to their thickheadedness.

If he had only taken a little more trouble, not to experiment with it in surgery himself, but to see that somebody else did so, then the whole credit of anæsthesia would have belonged to him. He would have gone straight to the top of the list without question. But he did not do it, and his idea remained stillborn, which explains his lowly place in the merit order.

Crawford W. Long (1815-1878) is another pioneer who could easily have held a much higher place. He had only himself to blame. Like Hickman he was a country general practitioner. Like Hickman he wanted to relieve pain in the infrequent small operations which came his way. But unlike Hickman he knew about the ether parties, and had taken part in them. So had some of his patients. He also knew that small injuries were not felt during ether intoxication.

One of his patients, Mr. James Venable, wanted a sebaceous cyst removing. But he did not want the inevitable pain which even a small operation like this would cause. It happened that Long had supplied him with ether before this, so when Long suggested that he inhale ether for the removal of the cyst his mind was quite receptive. The procedure was nothing new to him. The operation was performed on March 30th, 1842, and was not only successful but painless. Long charged him the very moderate fee of two dollars, with 25 cents extra for the ether. This was the first known, certain and premeditated case of surgical anæsthesia in the history of the world.

Long continued to use ether at infrequent intervals for some years and collected a small list of cases. But, and this is the strange thing about it, he never reported them, never took any steps whatever to make known this extraordinary and revolutionary, but successful, idea of surgery without pain. Not until ether anæsthesia had become a world-wide *fait accompli* through the exertion of others did Long put forward his claims to priority over Morton and Wells.

His proofs were beyond doubt. The receipted bill for Mr. Venable's operation, together with sworn statements from the patient and the spectators, were enough to settle the matter beyond argument. The only remaining uncertainty is why Long did not report his cases sooner. He, unlike most of the other pioneers, can certainly not be accused of precipitancy or undue haste. He was a truthful, modest man—either pathologically modest or unimaginative to a degree. Surely very little vision was required to realise what a tremendous discovery he had made. But only in 1849 did he write "An account of the first use of sulphuric ether by inhalation as an anæsthetic in surgical operations" in the *Southern Medical and Surgical Journal*.

Long's place in the ranking order is low simply because of this extra-ordinary reticence. He was beyond doubt the first successful practical anæsthetist the world had ever seen, antedating Wells by two years and Morton by four, but, if it had not been for the efforts of these two men, anæsthesia would have died, as it was born, with Crawford W. Long.

Simpson (1811-1870), who ended his days as Sir James Young Simpson, Bart., comes next. There was no originality about him—not as regards anæsthesia, anyway. He had nothing to do with its introduction, which was entirely due to others. His mind was receptive enough, though, and he welcomed the new idea at once. He began to use ether in his obstetric practice as soon as the news reached him, and liked it. But he did not consider it was perfect, and his enquiring mind soon began to look round for something better. He deserves every credit for this. Moreover he tested drugs on himself, helped by his assistants Keith and Matthew Duncan. So he was not deficient in courage. The amount of this work, however, was not large. Nothing like the vast amount of work done later by Sir Benjamin Ward Richardson, which led to very little of permanent value, and nothing like the long and painstakingly detailed work which Davy had put into nitrous oxide.

Simpson tested, by the rough and ready but practical method of inhalation, Dutch liquid, acetone, nitric ether, benzin and iodoform vapour, but without success. Also chloride of hydrocarbon, aldehyde and bisulphuret of carbon. Then at the suggestion of David Waldie, a Liverpool chemist, he and his experimental co-guinea-pigs tried chloroform, or perchloride of formyle, as it was then called. They found that it worked and worked well.

John Marshall[1] stated that the specimen of chloroform used by Simpson on the 4th November was sent to him by the late Professor Thomas Graham from his laboratory at University College. But Waldie's claim is supported by Simpson himself. Not that Simpson ever acknowledged this invaluable help as generously as he should have done. Waldie was one of the few men then living who knew anything about the drug, and without his suggestion Simpson would never have heard of it, for it was then a chemical curiosity only. In some of his writings he makes a perfunctory mention of Waldie, in others he does not—somewhat scurvy treatment, in my opinion.

Waldie's own account of the affair was published in a small pamphlet:—[2]

To the best of my knowledge, from the result of many inquiries, it seems to have been introduced into this country as a medicinal agent first in Liverpool, where indeed, in the form of a spirituous solution, it has been more known than in any other part of the country, and from which, I believe the knowledge of its therapeutic properties has extended. About the year 1838 or 1839 a prescription was brought to the Apothecaries' Hall, Colquitt Street, one ingredient of which was chloric ether. No substance being known there of that name, having the properties of that with which the mixture had been previously prepared, Dr. Brett, then the Company's chemist, in investigating the subject, found, in the United States Dispensatory, the formula for its preparation, and prepared some. Its properties pleased some of the medical men, particularly Dr. Formby, by whom it was introduced into practice in this town. After coming to take charge of the Company's laboratories, I found that the method of preparation yielded a product which was not of uniform strength, and sometimes of disagreeable flavour. Accordingly I altered the process, by separating and purifying the chloroform, and dissolving it in pure spirit, by which a product of uniform strength and sweet flavour was always obtained. Thus prepared, it is much superior to specimens I have seen of London manufacture. Those members of the profession who are in the habit of using it, prefer it greatly to sulphuric ether, as possessing all its remedial value, and being very much more agreeable. The vapour of the so-called chloric ether seems to have been tried as a substitute for sulphuric ether in February or March last (a reference to Furnell or Holmes Coote), but without very satisfactory results, which, indeed, could scarcely be expected, unless the vapour of alcohol possessed the same properties, it being composed principally of alcohol. When in Scotland in October last, Dr. Simpson introduced the subject to me, inquiring if I knew of anything likely to answer. Chloric ether was mentioned during the conversation, and being well acquainted with its composition, and with the volatility, agreeable flavour, and medicinal properties of chloroform, I recommended him to try *it*, promising to prepare some after my return to Liverpool, and send it to him. Other engagements and various impediments, prevented me from doing this so soon as I should have wished, and in the meantime Dr. Simpson having procured some in Edinburgh, obtained the results which he communicated to the Medico-Chirurgical Society of Edinburgh on the 10th of November.

I found later that my opinion about Simpson's treatment of Waldie was shared by Waldie himself. In a letter from him to John Abraham, a Liverpool chemist, written on July 8th, 1870,[3] two months after Simpson's death, he said:

"Though I never said much on the subject I was never satisfied with the recognition my share in the matter got, because I could never admit that the acknowledgment made by Dr. Simpson was at all adequate. He did as little as he could possibly do, and the statement he made was not a fair one. . . . Pity that the place (Waldie's laboratory) had been burned down at the time of Simpson's enquiries, I should in all probability have made the discovery myself."

Simpson's first and crucial experiments were made at his own home on the 4th November, when he and several others chloroformed themselves round the dinner table. Mrs. Agnes Thompson, who as Miss Petrie, was one of the experimenters and the first woman to inhale chloroform, lived until January, 1914.

Simpson, like most of the others except Crawford Long, dashed enthusiastically into print at very short notice. Six days later he read a paper, referred to above by Waldie, in which he sang the praises of chloroform with an uncritical optimism which had no real foundation in his pitifully short experience. "I have found, however, one infinitely more efficacious than any of the others. I am enabled to speak most confidently of its superior anæsthetic properties, having now tried it upon upwards of thirty individuals." (!!)

The avenging Furies which punished the unfortunate Wells for his

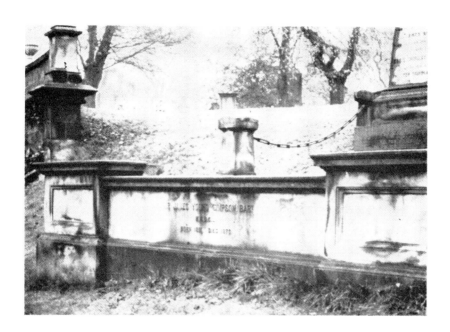

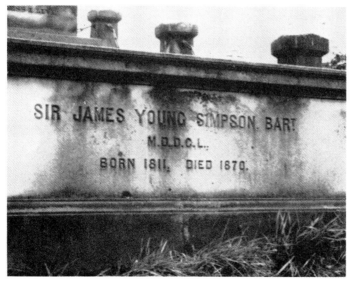

PLATE XXXI

Legend on back

PLATE XXXI

Grave of Sir James Y. Simpson in Warriston Cemetery, Edinburgh.

Photographs taken by the author on a wet, misty day when it was raining hard.

Lancet, 1870, May 14. 704. "Terrible are the accounts of his attacks of angina. They are only relieved by the accounts of his patience and piety, and by learning that in his own chloroform he got relief from one of his worst attacks."

Lancet, 1870, May 14. 716. Obituary notice. "At last Simpson, acting upon a hint supplied to him by Mr. Waldie, a chemist in Liverpool, made a series of experiments with chloroform, and so succeeded in assuring himself of its efficacy that he did not hesitate to proclaim it to the world as the long sought for yet finally discovered anæsthetic. Before making this announcement he had satisfied himself, at the cost of much labour and of many hundred pounds, that chloroform was open to no serious objection in competent hands."

This is mostly pure baloney. There are four mistakes in one short paragraph: 1, Waldie did not hint. He definitely suggested chloroform by name to Simpson; 2, A few casual, hasty experiments carried out round the dinner table are magnified to "much labour"; 3, The cost of a sample bottle of chloroform was certainly not "many hundred pounds"; 4, "Satisfied himself . . . that chloroform was open to no serious objection." As the news was made public six days after his first experiment, nothing was known, nothing could be known, at this stage, whether chloroform possessed any dangers or not.

Simpson will always be remembered for the work he did, without building a mythology around it.

Lancet, 1870, June 11. 854. A very charming and kindly tribute was paid to Sir James from the United States. At a meeting in Washington Dr. Storer of Boston proposed: "Whereas it is an instinctive and very natural desire among men to lament with those who are in affliction, and to mourn with those who weep, and whereas it has pleased the Giver of both mortal and eternal life to call unto Himself His good and faithful servant, known upon earth as Dr. James Y. Simpson, of Edinburgh, it is therefore

"Resolved: That in Dr. Simpson, American physicians recognise, not merely an eminent and learned Scotch practitioner, but a philanthropist whose love encircled the world; a discoverer who sought and found for suffering humanity, in its sorest need, a foretaste of the peace of heaven, and a devoted disciple of the only true Physician, our Saviour, Jesus Christ.

"Resolved: That in acknowledging for ourselves and our brethren the excellence of him who has gone, and in thus honouring his memory, we would tender to the members of his family in their sorrow our respectful sympathy.

"Resolved: That a copy of these resolutions be sent to the widow of Sir James Simpson, and to the British Minister resident at Washington, with the request to the latter that they may be transmitted by him to the several English medical journals, as a mark of the esteem felt in this country for the deceased."

The resolutions were seconded by Dr. William P. Johnston. Lady Simpson died on 17th June, six days after the publication of this thoughtful and gracious tribute in Britain, but the meeting was held on the 9th May, so that it is to be hoped that she received this delightful and comforting message in time.

A little later (*Lancet, 1870, July 9. 57*) a new appointment was made to the Chair of Midwifery at Edinburgh, left vacant by the death of Sir James. There were three candidates—Matthews Duncan, Keiller and A. R. Simpson. The two first named had all the qualifications, prestige and experience required. The latter had had little practice and little experience, but he had his uncle's popularity with the Town Council element which partially controlled the election, and he had the museum of speciments collected by Sir James over many years. So Simpson was duly appointed, and *The Lancet* had many critical things to say about it.

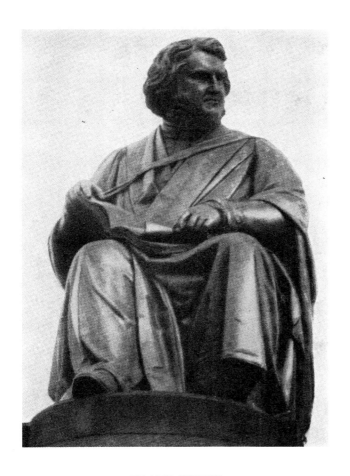

PLATE XXXII

Statue of Sir James Simpson, in Princes Street,
Edinburgh.

Photograph taken by the author, 1959.

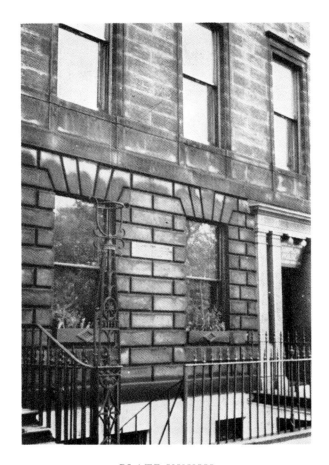

PLATE XXXIII

Sir James Simpson's house, 52 Queen Street,
Edinburgh.

Photograph taken by the author.

presumption with disgrace, drug addiction, madness, prison and suicide, evidently relented slightly so far as Morton was concerned. His punishment was limited to a long and rather undignified battle of words with Jackson, denial by many people of the priority and credit which was his just due, many promises of fame and reward which mostly failed to materialise, constant financial worries and an early death due to a cerebral hæmorrhage. Now the Furies had apparently gone off duty altogether. For the first time in the short history of anæsthesia fame and good fortune were immediately showered upon one of its pioneers—the one who had least need of them. He already had a great professional reputation, a professorship of honour and dignity, and a large and lucrative practice. But to him that hath shall be given, and Simpson died full of honours. He was also given a baronetcy at a time when the obstetrician's status was rather lower than it deserved to be—he had only just discarded the somewhat contemptuous title of man-midwife.

What had Simpson done to deserve all this? As already stated, he had really not done very much. A few random and cursory experiments with a drug suggested to him by somebody else gave him rapid, unexpected and undeservedly quick results. Further, he had, more than any of the others, a very large slice of good luck. His, or rather Waldie's, anæsthetic, chloroform, appeared at first sight to have all the virtues, to be without flaw and perfect. It was powerful, pleasant, portable, easy to give, convenient and cheap. It was non-inflammable and could be given in small rooms not far from a fire, a candle or a gas jet. Its advantages were so outstanding and overwhelming that Simpson launched it on the world with indecent haste, before he really knew anything about it at all. The casual and superficial nature of his work is well illustrated by his airy reference to "upwards of thirty individuals."

No, Simpson's outstanding service to anæsthesia was not his use of chloroform, that beautiful, easy and treacherous drug, but his energy as a propagandist. Pamphlet after pamphlet poured from his vituperative pen in defence of chloroform. He battled with the theologians on their own ground, delving deeply into the exact meanings of the Hebrew words in the Book of Genesis. Long and acrimonious were the controversies, but Simpson eventually won. Once more he was lucky, for he had an unexpected but very powerful ally on his side. After John Snow had given chloroform to Queen Victoria on April 7th, 1853, at the birth of Prince Leopold, and again on April 14th, 1857, at the birth of Princess Beatrice, the opposition died down. Such was the far-reaching influence of that strong-minded and very remarkable woman.

Simpson was selfish, in that he never gave proper credit to Waldie for his all-important suggestion, nor to his assistants, who had shared the risk of his experiments. He was also arrogant. The success of his new anæsthetic was so overwhelming that it rapidly superseded ether almost everywhere for the next twenty years or so. Chloroform became a popular synonym for anæsthesia itself, which was not surprising, for during this period chloroform *was* anæsthesia. This went to Simpson's head, and in some of his speeches and lectures he spoke as though he was the originator of anæsthesia itself.

He was by nature an enthusiast, which helped him enormously as a propagandist; but it is never easy for an enthusiast to keep a proper sense of proportion. Another of his inventions was acupressure, a method of checking hæmorrhage by pins instead of ligatures. This was thought by him to be one of the greatest advances ever made in surgery. It was in fact but a little thing and unimportant to a degree. It perished quickly, killed by the brutal ridicule of Syme, and the world did not lose much when it died.

His greatest work never came to full fruition. A little more luck and he would have anticipated the discoveries of a much greater man, Lister, and uncovered the secrets of clean surgery. His essay on Hospitalism represented a lot of painstaking work which only just missed a great result. He collected statistics from all over the country—this in the days when medical statistics were practically unknown. He found that the mortality of amputations had the following range:

	Number of cases	Size of hospital	Number of deaths	Death rate	Converted to percentages, more familiar to modern eyes
1	2089	Over 300 beds	855	1 in 2·4	40·9%
2	803	201-300	228	1 in 3·5	28·3%
3	1370	101-200	301	1 in 4·4	21·9%
4	761	26-100	134	1 in 5·6	17·6%
5	143	25 or less	20	1 in 7·1	14·0%
6	2098	in private or in single rooms	226	1 in 9·2	10·7%
	5264		1764	1 in 3	33·5%

It is easy enough to see now that dirty operations in private houses would be much less dangerous than dirty operations in big hospitals soaked and saturated with laudable pus and virulent pathogenes, but it was not so easy then. Simpson's work on this subject was far greater, more imaginative, more profound and more original than his work on chloroform, but who remembers it now?

An amusing incident concerning Simpson and his enthusiasms occurred in 1847. A long, complicated and very acrimonious dispute took place between him and Robert Lee, M.D., F.R.S., Lecturer in Midwifery at St. George's Hospital. The subject was the treatment of placenta prævia, and charges of incompetence and unreliable statistics were freely made on both sides. Dr. Lee fired his final broadside in the November 20th issue of *The Lancet* in the form of a violently libellous but devastatingly accurate prophecy:

"Probably there was never huddled together in so contracted a space . . . such a mass of glaring and mischievous errors; . . . I have great difficulty in comprehending how any man endowed with common sense, and the ordinary feelings of humanity, could have ventured to publish such a statement, and in such a manner deceive and mislead the inexperienced and unwary. I have felt it to be a duty which I owed to my professional brethren to expose these disgraceful and dangerous errors . . . my aim has been to prove, before the face of the profession, that the practice of tearing away the adherent placenta from the neck of the uterus, either by the hand, or by an iron or other instrument, is a murderous practice and . . . I am content to leave it to the profession to decide whether these things are or are not so? We shall see whether scientific *accoucheurs* abide by the old established rules of practice, and whether Dr. Simpson himself does not flee off to some new marvel, some fresh novelty, to attract public notoriety, and to cover his defeat in the battle of placenta prævia. . . ."

Rarely has any prophecy been so promptly fulfilled, for in the very next column is printed Simpson's classic article, *On a new anæsthetic agent, more efficient than sulphuric ether*!

It was Simpson's luck again that his best known and most spectacular contribution to science should be published on the same page as this savage attack. But Dr. Lee was not to be convinced, even when chloroform was in the full tide of its success. Knowing what he thought about Simpson this is hardly surprising. He might conceivably have accepted chloroform if somebody else had discovered it, but not from the hands of his *bête noire*. Can any good thing come out of Nazareth?

As late as 1853[4] he weighed in with another diatribe:

"Very soon after the discovery the author was astonished by its application to midwifery; and it was not difficult for him to foresee that rashness in its use would lead to most deplorable results and he regretted to find that he had not been mistaken. He had no doubt that the use of this noxious agent ought to be expelled from the practice of midwifery. 'In sorrow shalt thou bring forth children' was an established law of nature—an ordinance of the Almighty, as stated in the Bible."

Dr. Lee had evidently not read Simpson's theological pamphlets, or else he had not been convinced by them. "It was a most unnatural practice to destroy the consciousness of women during labour, the pains and sorrows of which exerted a most powerful and salutary influence upon their religious and moral character, and upon all their future relations in life."

He proceeded to relate 17 cases in which chloroform had been used with bad results—hearsay evidence surely, for in view of his very strong views on the iniquity of chloroform they could hardly have been his own cases. Nor would he alter his opinion. Dr. Snow, the acknowledged expert on anæsthesia, criticised most of the alleged bad effects on the grounds that some of them were *post hoc* and not *propter hoc*, while others came too late, long after the chloroform had been eliminated.

Dr. Gream said that Dr. Lee was determined to throw over everything that was novel merely because it was new. He (Dr. Gream) had strongly opposed chloroform, but had now modified his views. Mr. Ferguson said that he had seen no analogous cases in surgery to the seventeen cases reported by Dr. Lee. In any case the 17 were not all the cases in which chloroform had been used. It had probably been used in thousands.

But, no, nothing could shake Dr. Lee.

"In forceps cases . . . chloroform could produce nothing but mischief, for in all these cases consciousness was the great safeguard of the patient. No forceps cases were so unmanageable as those in which consciousness was lost from puerperal convulsions, where the patient could not be held in the same position for any length of time."

Simpson had many other critics besides Dr. Lee. Robert Barnes, another well known London obstetrician, took exception to his statistics, amongst other things.[5]

"We are commanded rather than recommended by Dr. Simpson to apathise our patients during the progress of natural labour. . . . What is it that emboldens Dr. Simpson to stigmatise nineteen out of twenty . . . medical men as influenced by indolence and apathy, by caprices and prejudices? . . . It has been said that facts are stubborn things; Dr. Simpson has shown them to be singularly pliable. . . . I do not condemn, *prima facie*, the use of ether or chloroform in midwifery, but I must first be convinced, by other arguments than Dr. Simpson has urged, that it is desirable, and that it is safe to use them. . . . The question is not to be decided . . . by wanton abuse of medical practitioners, by inconclusive arguments reared on a few imperfect and doubtful facts, and those facts wrested from their legitimate applications; by false analogy, bad arithmetic, and statistics run wild; however conclusive they may be to the judgement, and agreeable to the taste of the Edinburgh professor of midwifery."

Other people attacked his methods and the instruments he designed. Isaac Irons[6] says:

"To Dr. Simpson we owe the invention of the dangerous weapon called the uterine sound or poker; pessaries which have justly been designated infernal and impaling uterine machines, to cure retroversions which never existed; . . . to him we owe the hysterotome, for slitting open the os uteri, to cure sterility; . . . To Dr. Simpson we owe the attempt to revive the brutal practice of turning in cases of distortion of the pelvis; of attempting to substitute the Cæsarian (sic) operation for the induction of premature labour. . . . To him we owe the attempt to subvert the established practice in placental presentation by extraordinary statistic tables; and lastly we owe to the genius of the Professor of midwifery in the University of Edinburgh, the baby-sucker!"

(This was a reference to an idea of Simpson's that a leather sucker attached to a cord might be stuck on to the baby's head in order to provide less damaging traction than the blades of the forceps.)

Samuel Ashwell, late obstetric physician to Guy's Hospital, was dead against the use of chloroform in natural labour,[7] and also criticised Simpson's theological arguments.

"Dr. Simpson refers, in his pamphlet on the religious objections which have been urged to chloroform, to the first operation ever performed—namely the extraction of the rib of Adam, as having been executed while our progenitor was in a state of sopor, which the professor learnedly argues was similar to the anæsthesia of chloroform. . . . Putting aside the impiety of making Jehovah an operating surgeon, and the absurdity of supposing that anæsthesia would be necessary in His hands, Dr. Simpson surely forgets that the deep sleep of Adam took place before the introduction of pain into the world, during his state of innocence!"

Robert Barnes[8] returns to the attack on the ground that too much is claimed for chloroform. It is said to decrease the pains when they are too strong and to increase them when they are too weak. . . . He also protests against the unfair treatment of Dr. Meggison after the first death under chloroform. Dr. Simpson says that he killed her by pouring brandy and water into her mouth when she was unconscious—by drowning her, in fact. . . .

"It is surely riding a hobby somewhat too hard, when all its mishaps are saddled on those who use it. . . . If anyone follows Dr. Simpson's advice let them not hope that Dr. Simpson will come forward to protect them. Before the result of twelve cases were known to him he had already drawn the conclusion that it ought to be resorted to in every case of natural parturition."

Dr. G. T. Gream,[9] surgeon *accoucheur* to Queen Charlotte's Hospital, was opposed, at this date, to chloroform in labour, although he later changed his mind.

"Dr. Simpson . . . considers, that in the few cases in which he has exhibited chloroform he has been enabled to gain such experience as will allow him to publish to the world that it may be employed in all cases of natural as well as artificial delivery. . . . If chloroform was exhibited at Newcastle to an improper subject, the justification rests in the repeated commendation of it by Dr. Simpson as an agent in all instances. . . . The arguments (in Simpson's article) are too futile to call for contradiction; it is sufficient to notice, that Dr. Simpson has failed to prove that the cause of death . . . was any other than the direct result of this most dangerous agent."

The cause of most of this trouble was a report by Simpson about nine obstetrical cases in which chloroform was used. He argued that pain in itself was dangerous—or could be—and destructive. He supported this argument with some figures alleged to show that the mortality increased in direct proportion to the duration of the labour.

The robust virulence and rudeness of the opposition certainly explains why Simpson fought with the gloves off. It also shows that the theologians were not the only opponents whom he had to crush with the hammer blows of his logic! Much may be forgiven to a man who has the exasperating task of dealing with people who are utterly impervious to new ideas. That is not to say that all new ideas are good. They may be better than the old or they may not. The chances are about even. But a blank refusal to entertain them at all is very different from a reasoned and reasonable caution.

Many of the early pamphlets on chloroform possessed this caution, which in itself is open to no objection—it is in fact desirable, if only to offset the over-optimistic claims of the enthusiasts—Simpson himself, and Syme, for example.

Charles Thomas Jackson (1805-1880), the last of the pioneers, really does not deserve to be in the list at all. He did not have the idea of anæsthesia in the first place. All he did was to try and cash in upon it when it proved to be successful. He did no work upon it himself, and there is little evidence that he ever used ether at all, although he wrote a book about it.[10] He did not even take the trouble to see an anæsthetic given until five weeks after Ether Day.[11] It is almost incredible that a man who claimed, or was about to claim, an important part in such an obviously revolutionary idea, should take so little interest in its development. It tends to prove that his part in the whole affair was very small indeed, and that it only assumed importance in his eyes when it showed signs of being successful, and possibly lucrative.

On the 21st November, 1846, Dr. J. Mason Warren removed a tumour of the thigh; at long last Jackson condescended to be present to see 'his' discovery used, "and this was the first operation upon a patient, under the influence of ether, which that gentleman had witnessed."[12]

Any services he may have rendered in advocacy or publicity were purely for the purpose of personal aggrandisement. He needed no courage, for he did no work on anæsthesia himself, either theoretical or practical. He was lucky, in that his sole contribution to anæsthesia, his suggestion to Morton that ether might be used instead of nitrous oxide, happened to be a good one. And it is quite possible that Morton knew this already.

But that is not quite fair. Jackson was not a stupid man; he was a scientist with a good brain, and he did make a useful suggestion to the effect that during ether anæsthesia a safety lamp should be used if light was wanted near the mouth. Self-assertive and pushful he was, for he tried to transfer the credit of the whole thing from Morton, who had done all the work and risked all the criticism and ridicule, to himself, who had done so little. But he was at the same time timid, for he sold out his share of Morton's patent rights (which never became effective) at the moment when the success of the venture seemed doubtful.

He was by way of being a professional purloiner of other people's inventions, for he had done the same thing before, notably in the case of Morse's telegraph. The kindest thing that can be said of him is that his conduct was probably due to the early stages of the insanity which finally condemned him to death in a mental hospital; to a fixed idea that he, and he alone, was the originator and inventor of any idea brought forward by anybody with whom he had been in contact. Jackson's character has been well summarised by Raper:[13]

"He had a well-trained, well-stocked, well-disciplined brain, but there was a sick spot in it. Having worked so hard and so successfully to master science, he appears to have concluded that if any great discoveries were to be made, he was the logical and inevitable one to make them . . . to see Morton, an 'ignoramus' (Jackson's word) in scientific matters, or Wells, a mere dentist, get all the credit for the greatest scientific discovery of the age was too much for him. He did everything he could to keep them from it. As his frustrations grew, signs of pathologic obsession multiplied in him. He laid claim not only to the discovery of anæsthesia . . . "

W. A. Comstock of Boston[14] has a very apt and conclusive reply to Jackson's contemptuous attitude towards Morton. "If it be true that this Mr. Morton was as ignorant as he is declared to be, not only of all physiological laws, but of the very existence of sulphuric ether, why did Dr. Jackson select him as the one whom he would induce to test a discovery of this nature?" Why, indeed?

Such were the men who laid the foundation stones. A mixed crowd, but an interesting one. There is no point in recapitulating their experiences in detail. That has been done before, and done well. They were very human and had their faults—just like us. Selfishness was one of them. Morton never acknowledged the help he received from Wells' previous work on nitrous oxide. Simpson never acknowledged his debt to Waldie, without whose aid he would never have heard of chloroform, which was then only a laboratory curiosity.

But we might have done exactly the same. . . .

REFERENCES

[1] *Lancet* (1890), Aug. 2. 243.
[2] *Lancet* (1847), Dec. 25. 687.
[3] *Lancet* (1933), Dec. 30. 1515.
[4] *Lancet* (1853), Dec. 24. 608.
[5] *Lancet* (1847), Dec. 25. 677.
[6] *Lancet* (1851), Sept. 20. 284.
[7] *Lancet* (1848), Mar. 11. 291.
[8] *Lancet* (1848), April 22. 442.
[9] *Lancet* (1848), Feb. 26. 228.
[10] *A Manual of Etherization.* Boston. 1861.
[11] *Lancet* (1847), April 3. 354. John Gardner.
[12] *Boston med. surg. J.* (1847), May 26. Vol. 36. 335.
[13] Howard Riley Raper (1945). *Man against Pain.* 324 pages. New York. Prentice-Hall, Inc.
[14] *Boston med. surg. J.* (1847), July 14. Vol. 36. 482.

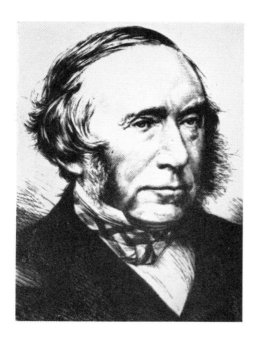

PLATE XXXIV

Brit. med. J., 1870, July 2. 21. James Syme. Born Nov. 7, 1799. Died June 26, 1870. At one time in partnership with Liston, until they quarrelled. He ran a private hospital, as he could not get on to the staff of the Royal Infirmary as long as Liston was there. In 1834 Liston went to London and Syme was appointed surgeon to the Infirmary. He did the first amputation at the hip joint. He removed the clavicle, ligatured the subclavian artery, and designed Syme's amputation. He also ligatured the internal iliac artery. A copious writer on surgical subjects. On Feb. 13, 1848, became surgeon to University College Hospital. Resigned on May 10 and went back to Edinburgh. He was pugnacious, combative, daring, argumentative and dogmatic. Also unscrupulous. Primarily an operating surgeon, in which he was cool, dexterous and original, if not brilliant. A good teacher on new cases, but his students did not get the chance to follow them up. He paid £300 a year to his predecessor as Professor in order to induce him to resign. He probably returned to Scotland because he was 50, was long used to being a surgical autocrat, and because he missed his friends (and enemies).

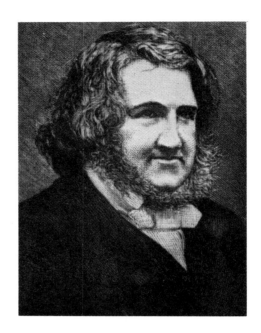

PLATE XXXV

Brit. med. J., 1896, Oct. 17. 1141. James Young Simpson, born 7th June, 1811, at Bathgate, Scotland. Qualified 1830. Professor of Midwifery, Edinburgh, in 1840, at the age of 29. Died 6th May, 1870. Buried in Warriston Cemetery, Edinburgh.

In 1865 he introduced acupressure, a method of hæmostasis by pins instead of ligatures. In 1867 (*Lancet, Nov. 2. 546*) he denied Lister's priority in the antiseptic method and stated that others had used phenol since 1865. He claimed that pyæmia disappeared from wards where his acupressure was used, without phenol. He first used chloroform on Nov. 4, 1847.

CHAPTER 8

THE SCOTTISH CHLOROFORM LEGEND.
SYME AND SIMPSON AS PRACTICAL ANÆSTHETISTS

"One can't believe impossible things."
"I daresay you haven't had much practice," said the Queen. "When I
was your age, I always did it for half an hour a day. Why, sometimes I've
believed as many as six impossible things before breakfast."
—LEWIS CARROLL, *Through the Looking-glass.*

ENTHUSIASTIC and successful users of chloroform like Surgeon-major
Lawrie of Hyderabad regarded Syme's method of anæsthesia with
an almost religious veneration, as a revelation to which nothing
could be added and from which nothing could be taken away. It was
something infallible, unalterable, which could not be shaken by facts
or rebutted by evidence. It was as the laws of the Medes and Persians.

The dogmatism of Simpson and Syme, founded as it was on a base
far too small to support the superstructure that was built upon it, led
directly to the creation of a legend which persisted for many decades—
that chloroform, which was known to be dangerous anywhere else in the
world, was perfectly safe when given in Scotland, and later, in Hyderabad.

I always had great difficulty in believing this extraordinary myth,
either before or after breakfast. Like Alice, perhaps I hadn't had enough
practice. But I also thought that it would be impossible at this date,
many years after all the founders of the legend were dead, to get any
evidence either for or against it. But a certain amount of evidence did
turn up, after a long and detailed study of old copies of the medical
journals, and it was even possible to form a fairly accurate judgment of
the flimsy grounds on which the legend was based—even a moderately
reliable estimate of the number of operations performed by Syme.

This surgeon gave a lecture on chloroform in 1855,[1] or rather part
of a lecture, for he did not consider anæsthesia as of sufficient importance
or complexity to devote a whole hour to it. The script of the lecture can
be read aloud slowly in less than ten minutes. He certainly claimed
success, for he said that he had been using it "almost daily", which is his
nearest approach to statistics. He said that he had never had a death
from it, though, like many others, he reported one in another part of
the hospital. This he regarded apparently as of no importance, because

it did not come under his own eye. Would he have thought the same if the patient had been Mrs. Syme?

Beyond this, with a modesty which was very rare in him, he claimed nothing. All he had done, he said, was to follow the example of Dr. Simpson. It was not until about ten years later that the truculent Syme quarrelled with Simpson and tore up in public one of the latter's pamphlets, which led to an almighty row.

So the Edinburgh method of using chloroform, which had a tremendous influence on anæsthesia for fifty years or more, and which put up a granite-like resistance against a mounting accumulation of adverse facts, really originated from Simpson. It was popularised and made into an article of faith by Syme, who, as the leading operating surgeon in Scotland, naturally had more chance of doing this. Obstetricians like Simpson, however eminent, were not in those days operating gynæcologists to any extent, as they are today. The vagina was not at that time obsolete as a mode of delivery in difficult cases, for a Cæsarean section meant almost certain death for the mother. Ramsbotham in 1841 gave the Cæsarean figures for the British Isles as 30, with 27 deaths. Robert Barnes as late as 1871, just at the beginning of the Listerian era, said that the mortality of Cæsarean section in Britain was 84%.[2] And the few resolute men who practised ovariotomy as a last resort in desperate cases which were being crushed to death by their enormous cysts were contemptuously known as "belly rippers". Cases are recorded in which the cyst and its contents weighed more than the patient from which it was removed.

One is apt to assume, therefore, that Simpson, as the originator of a persistent and widely accepted tradition, must have been a wonderful anæsthetist himself, in spite of the known fact that he was generally occupied with the other end of the patient. Was this really so? What actual evidence exists after all these years for Simpson's competence as an anæsthetist? A little, and what there is is not at all good. But he shall speak for himself, about his own death on the table in 1870,[3] three months before his own death.

"Mr. Brotherston of Alloa took the patient into the small village hospital and requested me to be present when he operated. On Feb. 5th I chloroformed the patient with a single layer of towel over the nose and mouth, leaving the eyes exposed. When Mr. Brotherston made his first cutaneous incision, the patient moved so much that he stopped for a brief time, till I put the patient more deeply under the effects of the anæsthetic. . . . Mr. Brotherston . . . was introducing his hand with the view of turning out the ovarian mass, when patient vomited suddenly and profusely. Immediately the eyes opened; the pupils were preternaturally dilated; the face looked pallid; and the respiration which had never been affected by the chloroform so as to have the least noise or stertor in it, seemed arrested. Instantly artificial respiration was set on foot, and the tongue pulled forward. Deep spontaneous respiration then occurred several times in succession, and I deemed at the moment that the patient was out of danger; but a second collapse occurred, which terminated in death, all means of resuscitation proving unavailing.

No disease was found post-mortem except that the ovarian tumour was cancerous. It is quite clear, after reading Sir James' own account, that, despite his 22 years' experience since he first introduced chloroform, he had no idea at all how to give an anæsthetic, no more idea than the student or hospital porter to whom he usually delegated this unimportant job.

The patient was obviously, from his own description, never under at all. She moved on incision sufficiently to stop the operation altogether for a time, she vomited on exploration and she opened her eyes. In fact this patient, for an abdominal operation, admittedly very rare in those days, was no more under than Hannah Greener was when her toe-nail was removed, and she died, no doubt, for this very reason. It is very unlikely that she died from inhaling vomit, for the face was pallid after the vomiting rather than cyanosed. Also the post-mortem would have revealed this, if it had happened. Simpson labours the obvious fact that there was no overdosage, judged by the breathing. It was hardly necessary to mention this, in view of the other evidence—of movements and vomiting.

Simpson went on to say:

"In the first paper which I published on chloroform in the *Edinburgh Monthly Journal of Medical Science*, for December, 1847, I stated that the drug, if given in too great or too long does would doubtless produce serious consequences, and even death; and at the same time I expressed the hope that its great potency would be one great safeguard against its abuse. . . . Since that period I have administered it myself, or been present when it was administered, in several thousands of instances.

His statistics are as vague and sketchy as those of his disciple Syme! But there is a much graver charge against Sir James than that of being a bad anæsthetist and a woolly-minded statistician. He goes on to say . . . "but have not seen its employment terminate in death before the occurrence of the preceding unhappy case." Unfortunately, this is quite simply not true. Dr. Roberts of Edinburgh had a chloroform death prior to dental extractions in 1855.[4] He sent his son running for help to Professor Simpson, who lived close by, and the Professor arrived in less than five minutes.

Could Sir James possibly have forgotten this? It is not easy to forget such a tragic case, even if you don't keep anæsthetic records, as he obviously did not. He was called in during an emergency, in a frantic hurry, to a healthy woman of thirty-six, who died whilst being chloroformed for the removal of four easy front teeth. The operation, such as it was, had not begun, and the patient was almost certainly dead when he got there, but he spent a long time (an hour and a quarter) in strenuous efforts at resuscitation, which failed. He finally took part in the autopsy and signed the post-mortem report. There was plenty to impress it on his memory, not least the fact that it happened very close to his own home. Could he ever pass that dentist's house again without being reminded of the tragedy caused by the drug which he had himself introduced? He was not senile at the time, being only 44. He was only 58 when he wrote about his own death on the table fifteen years later. So his memory should have been normal.

This dramatic proof that the Edinburgh dogma of the harmlessness of chloroform was wrong ought to have made an indelible impression on the mind of its discoverer and originator. Did he suppress it deliberately because he had not, in this case, given the anæsthetic himself? But his own words were, "I have administered it myself or been present when it was administered in several thousands of instances," so he cannot have meant to refer only to personal anæsthetics.

The remaining alternative is that he excluded it because he was not actually present at the administration, but only during the fruitless attempts to revive an already dead patient. If he did this, without mentioning the case *en passant*, it savours of very sharp practice, in fact, of actual deceit, in suppressing awkward facts in order to preserve the reputation of his beloved chloroform and the sanctity of his own dogma. Syme at least was honest enough to mention a chloroform death which he knew about, but at which he was not personally present, although how he reconciled this death with his dogma of perfect safety is beyond the comprehension of any ordinary person.

But Simpson's failure to mention such a case as this at all is even more difficult to understand, and it takes a lot of explaining away. His statement made in 1870 is quite definite; "I have . . . not seen its employment terminate in death before the occurrence of the preceding unhappy case," i.e. the ovariotomy. It is, of course, possible to make this technically, legally true, though actually false, by splitting hairs. For Simpson did not actually see the chloroform used in Dr. Roberts's case; but no one knew better than he did that it had been used a few minutes before his arrival.

Consider your verdict, ladies and gentlemen. I have given you the facts. To save you the trouble of looking up the original references I attach a summary of Sir James's comments on the ovariotomy death and the full report of the dental case. I have not consciously omitted anything of importance and have not distorted anything, as far as I know. In any case my abstract can always be compared with the originals. Syme's lecture is also worth quoting in full here—the whole of anæsthesia in ten minutes!—with John Snow's reply to it, and some comments on both of them. Syme and Snow were the protagonists of two irreconcilable schools of thought—the slap-happy, slosh-it-on-regardless method and the cautious, find-out-something-about-it and go carefully approach. The antagonism between them flared up into open warfare later in the century, when Lawrie's Hyderabad Commission got to work.

Simpson commented on his death on the table:

"Chloroform appears capable of destroying life in two ways—namely, (1) by asphyxia, and (2) by syncope. Death by asphyxia can generally, if not always, be averted by at once arresting the inhalation of the drug whenever the breathing becomes noisy or stertorous—states which, as already mentioned, never occurred with the preceding patient. Syncope, or sudden stoppage of the heart, is doubtless far less under control, and has apparently formed the principal cause of the fatal issue in almost all the cases in which patients have perished when under the use of chloroform. . . . But are all such cases of syncope which take place during operation . . . the result of the action of the chloroform which happens to be used at the time? For . . . before the introduction of anæsthetics, patients sometimes died from syncope upon the operating table, both immediately before and after the operation was commenced, and under conditions and circumstances which in modern times, when anæsthetics are almost universally used, would be not unnaturally described and regarded as deaths from chloroform. Formerly—such sudden deaths . . . do not seem to have been looked upon as matters of moment . . . they were simply regarded as inevitable accidents. . . . "

He describes ten of these deaths, one of which is particularly interesting, as it had such a profound influence over the future of chloroform.

"Case VII.—After discovering the anæsthetic effects of chloroform in November, 1847, I tested it in a case of tooth-pulling, but required to wait eight days before I had an opportunity of using it, in the hospital or elsewhere, in any surgical operations. A few days, however, after its discovery, a hernia, which had been strangulated for a few hours, was brought into the Infirmary, and Professor Miller thought it a case demanding operative interference, and one in which chloroform should be tried; but I could not be found in time for the purpose of giving it, and the patient was operated on without any anæsthetic."

It is not stated why ether was not used in this case.

"Professor Miller had only proceeded the length of dividing the skin, when the patient fainted, and died with the operation unfinished. If the chloroform had happened to be used, and this fatal syncope had occurred while the patient was under its action, the whole career of the new anæsthetic would have been at once arrested."

An interesting thought, and probably perfectly correct. The whole history of anæsthesia would have been different. Hannah Greener and hundreds of others would not have died when they did; the Hyderabad Commission would not have taken place, and people would have been compelled to learn how to give ether half a century sooner than they did . . . but all these things did not happen.

Death from Chloroform in Edinburgh. [5]
Dr. Roberts.

The sudden death of a lady, while under my care for the extraction of some teeth, having been reported in several of the journals as a case of "Death from chloroform," and having created a considerable sensation in the public mind, I consider it necessary to communicate the particulars of that unfortunate case, so that the profession may be enabled to judge as to the cause of the association of circumstances which brought about the fatal result.

Mrs. H—, aged 36 years, tall and rather delicate in appearance, called at 3 p.m. at my house, on Tuesday the 30th October last, accompanied by her husband, for the purpose of having the four lower incisor teeth extracted. With the intention of dissuading her from the use of chloroform, I remarked that the operation would be very simple, as the roots were single and by no means firm; but she replied, "Oh, but I must have chloroform. You have given it to me before and you must give it to me now." Her husband expressed no wish in the matter; and as I had administered chloroform to her on *four* previous occasions during the last twelve months, without any unusual effect, and as I was aware that her medical attendant in the country gave it to her during her *accouchement*, some months previous to her first visit, I consented to its employment on this occasion also.

While preparing to sit down in the operating chair, she said, "Have you heard of that case of death from chloroform which occurred lately in my neighbourhood, while a person was having a tooth extracted?" and again, when seated, she observed, "I feel rather nervous." My son assisted me in administering, in the usual way, the chloroform, which was the preparation of Messrs. Duncan and Flockart (sic). Mrs. H— had only taken about nine or ten inspirations, obtaining but the partial influence of a quantity short of a drachm and a half poured out from the bottle, and inhaling it for a space of time certainly less than a minute, when she said, "You must not operate until I am quite insensible"; and again, "I am not over yet, you must give me more—I am not over yet"; and *immediately, even while speaking,* she gave a convulsive start, and with a stertorous respiration, and with the eyes and mouth open, sunk to the floor.

The suddenness of this attack, the expression of the countenance, and the attitude, altogether so different from anything which I had ever witnessed from chloroform, although I had up to that time on my register 2,096 cases, in which I had operated with the use of chloroform, immediately alarmed me and I instantly desired my son to run for Professor Simpson, whose house is close at hand, in the meantime doing all that I could think of to resuscitate the patient; and as Dr. Simpson was fortunately at home, he came to my assistance, accompanied by Dr. Priestly, in less than five minutes from the time that the accident had happened. The means employed were pulling forward the tongue and keeping up artificial respiration; and as the face was greatly congested, bleeding was attempted, but not more than six or seven ounces could be procured. Galvanism was applied alternatively with artificial respiration, but produced no permanent benefit. After artificial respiration had been carried on for some time, repeated spontaneous inspirations were remarked, but at no time more frequent than five in the minute. The pulsations of the radial artery were at first not sensible, but, while the artificial breathing was going on, they became more distinct, and the livid appearance of the face in a great measure disappeared. The same improvement was also noticed when the galvanic current excited the muscles of respiration, which at first gave hopes of resuscitation. But, occurring as they did, more than once, ultimately declined, and after one hour and a quarter (4.20 p.m.) of the most energetic exertions (especially on the part of Dr. Simpson), the case was reluctantly abandoned as hopeless, life being manifestly extinct.

The following is the post-mortem examination, which was made twenty-eight hours after death by Drs. Simpson, Peddie and Priestly, along with my son and myself:—

Post-mortem examination of Mrs. H—, twenty-eight hours after death:— The general appearance of the body presented nothing unusual. The deep livid colour of the integument of the head and neck, and the injection of the conjunctivæ, which were observable at the time of death, had in a great measure disappeared.

On laying open the abdominal walls, the organs contained in that cavity were found, in most respects, healthy. The capillaries of the intestines were, however, distended with blood, giving to the convolutions of the bowels a more than usually deep-red colour.

The liver, too, was firmly adherent by the whole of its convex surface to the diaphragm, by old lymphy exudation, but when cut through, its substance revealed no other morbid change.

The uterus was healthy, and its appendages healthy.

In the dissection of the thorax, the lungs did not appear more than ordinarily congested, except posteriorly, where they were of a deeper colour, and contained more blood; this was, doubtless, the result of a post-mortem circumstance.

When the pericardium was laid open, the heart was found preternaturally small in comparison with the conformation of the body; the right side was flaccid and full of blood, while the left side was comparatively firm and contracted. On dividing the descending vena cava, a quantity (probably six or eight ounces) of dark, half-coagulated blood escaped from its tributaries, and from the right auricle.

The extreme thinness of the walls of the right auricle and ventricle were remarked when they were laid open; in fact, in no portion of the muscular substance of the right ventricle did the thickness exceed one-half of the normal proportions, and its component tissue was soft and lacerable.

Both right auricle and ventricle were gorged with dark blood, and the valves belonging to both cavities were healthy.

The left ventricle was contracted, and little blood remained in either ventricle or auricle of this side. The muscular parietes were thinner than usual, but the difference was less marked than on the right side.

Under the microscope, the muscular fibres of the right side of the heart, more especially of the ventricle, were much altered in appearance. The transverse striæ were indistinct, or had disappeared entirely in some portions, while fatty granules were everywhere observable, arranged in lines, along the direction of the fibres.

The same state was found to be present, but in a less degree, in the muscular tissue of the left ventricle; here, however, the fatty particles were few and scattered, and the transverse markings, for the most part, distinct.

The vessels of the brain were turgid with blood, but beyond this, the cerebral organ appeared healthy.

(Signed) J. Y. Simpson, A. Peddie, W. O. Priestly.

To these statements I have only to add, that I have been informed Mrs. H—'s father died some years since of disease of the heart, being found dead in his chair.

Queen Street, Edinburgh, Nov. 23, 1855.

None of the then standard explanations fitted this case. It was not operative shock, because the operation was never started. It was not idiosyncrasy, because the same patient had had chloroform repeatedly without incident. It was not overdosage because she was never unconscious. She died while she was still talking. Even Sir James' explanation of Hannah Greener's death did not apply—that she was drowned by brandy and water poured into her mouth. This was obviously not done. There is no mention of it in the very detailed account of the resuscitation procedures, and Sir James no doubt enquired about it. The only thing left was heart disease, which was looked for very carefully. The findings do not sound very convincing. Anyway her heart was good enough to take her safely through five other anæsthetics and a confinement.

The two points which escaped recognition were very significant. One was the element of fear and the other was the incredible, unbelievable fact that a person could be made drunk by giving him too little whisky. The element of fear in Mrs. H——'s case was something new to her. She had heard of a recent death and it alarmed her, with good reason.

An astonishingly large percentage of these early primary cardiac failures record the same thing. Even though its significance was not recognised, some such fact often crept into the case report in all innocence. For example, in one case a man was to be anæsthetised for an amputation of a toe.[6] After half an ounce of chloroform had been used he was still not under. The whole supply of chloroform was then exhausted, and more had to be sent for! The unfortunate man was kept waiting on the operating table for more than two hours before the second attempt was made. He then died like a shot rabbit in a few seconds. Just imagine his feelings during the apparently endless delay! The verdict was "died of chloroform properly (!) administered."

And now for Syme's ten minute lecture on the whole art and science of anæsthesia. Those who have spent years in obtaining the F.F.A. should appreciate this.

Lancet (1855), Jan. 20, 55. *Lectures on Clinical Surgery*, by James Syme, Esq., Professor of Clinical Surgery in the University of Edinburgh.[7]

LECTURE III

CHLOROFORM.

I have now to speak of some cases in which chloroform will be given as usual, in consequence of the pain otherwise attendant on the operation to be performed; but before the patients are brought in I may take this opportunity of saying a few words regarding the use of chloroform, as you see that fatal cases, I am sorry to say, still occur, and that the medical journals, consequently, express doubts as to the use of chloroform at all, or say that, if used, it must be only with the greatest caution. Chloroform is no doubt a very powerful agent, sufficient to destroy the strongest individual if employed freely enough. Its fatal effects were shown at an early period in the following way; a lecturer in London was illustrating its action upon a guinea-pig, which was placed under a glass jar with some of the anæsthetic; the professor in the eagerness of his discourse, left the animal too long under the jar, and it died. He explained to his audience the cause of the accident, but though the reasons he gave were satisfactory, yet an impression was made upon the public which was not soon effaced. In this respect, however, there is nothing peculiar to chloroform as a medicinal agent; opium, prussic acid, strychnia, etc., not only may, but often do, destroy life, through being used in overdoses. But the question is, may it be used, judiciously, so as to do the good without exposing the patient to the risk of the evil? It is said in London that it cannot; that the risk is so great that it is only justifiable to use it in case of operations accompanied with an extreme degree of pain, or where stillness on the part of the patient is essential to success, and that the greatest caution is required in its administration; here we say that, if used with moderate care, it is perfectly safe. It was in this theatre that chloroform was first administered in public, by Dr. Simpson, seven years ago; since then it has been almost daily given here, yet we have not had a fatal case. It is true that one solitary instance of death from chloroform has occurred in another part of the hospital, but that case has nothing to do with us; so far as my department is concerned, it might as well have been at Guy's Hospital, or in Kamschatka, or anywhere else; indeed, it so happened, that at the very time when that unfortunate event was taking place in another part of the establishment, I was myself performing an operation on a patient under chloroform in this theatre.

"Almost daily" for seven years. Didn't anybody keep any records of their work in those days? A few simple figures would be so helpful; not necessarily the alarming and formidable symbols with which statisticians today decorate all medical papers.

To surgeons accustomed to the old pre-anæsthetic custom of one short operating session a week for the whole hospital staff the spate of new work produced by painless surgery might well make three times a week seem almost daily. If this were the case the total number in seven years would be just over a thousand.

After the above was written a little piece of evidence turned up which confirmed my estimate very strongly. It clearly shows that Syme was, in fact, exaggerating when he used the vague expression "almost daily." Mr. Annandale, a young resident, who became one of Syme's successors as Professor of Clinical Surgery much later, after Lister went to London (Annandale was thirty-nine years younger than Syme) wrote a letter[8] giving the exact number of operations performed at the Edinburgh Royal Infirmary for the month of November, 1862.

His object was to point out the wealth of material which was available for students at that institution. The figures he gave were: Mr. Syme 13, Mr. Spence 8, Mr. Gillespie 3, Professor Miller 2. (These did not include 12 eye operations and a few minor cases. A total of 26 operations in a month for the whole staff gives an average of just over 300 a year; certainly a vast—probably six-fold—increase over the figures of the pre-anæsthetic era. But it was nothing out of the ordinary, as Mr. Annandale appeared to think. All other large hospitals had experienced the same increase. The operations at St. Bartholomew's Hospital in London totalled 340 for 1860.[9]

It will be noted that Syme had exactly the same amount of operative surgery as the other three surgeons put together—an average of about 150 a year, or three a week. So my estimate of a probable thousand in seven years was, in fact, surprisingly accurate. It should be realised that Syme was at the height of his fame at the relevant dates. In 1855, the date of his lecture, he was 56, and at the time of Annandale's letter he was sixty-three. He bestrode British surgery after the death of Robert Liston, as the acknowledged master of them all. The break in his career when he made his abortive attempt to migrate to London was far behind him (it was in 1848, just after Liston's death); the hemiplegia which led to his retirement did not take place until much later (1869).

So if we assume that his work remained more or less constant at the monthly number of operations reported by Mr. Annandale, which is probably over-estimating the total in his favour, his whole hospital experience of anæsthesia, in the 21 years from the introduction of chloroform until his resignation, would be just over three thousand.

But the fact remains that, at the time of this lecture, when he claimed absolute safety for chloroform and backed this preposterous claim with the full weight of his international reputation as a surgeon, his hospital experience was limited, after seven years, to a bare thousand cases. No doubt it seemed an enormous number to him—seven years successful use, when operating far more frequently than in the old days, and far more frequently than any of his Edinburgh colleagues. Perhaps it is no wonder that he thought he knew it all. But it was a very weak and very small foundation upon which to build a confident, infallible dogma.

But, in fairness to Syme—though it was really his fault, because he never mentions it in his lecture, something has been omitted from these calculations—his private work. He was referring—the wording makes it quite obvious—to his hospital cases only. The result was that I only thought of this addition to his total after writing this section—and had to rewrite it. Here, I am afraid, we are on less secure ground. I could find no details about the number of his private operations, so we have to fall back on guesswork. Intelligent guesswork, I hope, but still an estimate only, with no real evidence to support it.

Scotland was a poor country at that time, and sparsely populated, with a very few big-town exceptions, so the number of patients able to pay for private surgery would be limited. On the other hand Syme's reputation was so great that he doubtless took the lion's share of what there was, just as in hospital his operations far outnumbered those of the other surgeons. His fame would also attract patients from outside Scotland.

Suppose we assume that his private operations were equal in number to his hospital operations. I think this would be a generous estimate for nineteenth century conditions. That would mean that his total experience at the time of the lecture was about two thousand cases instead of one. A slightly better and broader foundation for his dogma, but still utterly inadequate and insufficient. His total experience until he retired from work, under this new estimate, would be six thousand.

The article on Anæsthesia in Holmes and Hulke's *System of Surgery*[10] was not written by an anæsthetist (Clover would have been the obvious man) but by Joseph, later Lord, Lister, who married Syme's daughter Agnes. In Part I of his article, which dates from 1861, he stated that Syme had given chloroform about five thousand times, which agrees fairly well with the above calculations. As Syme was Lister's father-in-law, the latter probably got the figure direct from him, for what it is worth.

Dr. Roberts, the Edinburgh dentist, who did keep a record of his cases, also had over two thousand cases without any fatality. His first death was his 2,097th chloroform case. No one has ever seriously accused chloroform of being responsible for more than about one death per thousand on the average—some estimates were half this mortality rate. A few unfortunates might have had more, but many people, aided by skill and luck, reported much larger numbers of cases without incident.

Hunter McGuire, a very successful user of chloroform in the American Civil War, reported about 13,000 cases without a death. He was chief surgeon to Stonewall Jackson's Army, was born in 1835 and died Sept. 19, 1900. But even he had a death under his own hands in 1882, a primary syncope in which the heart stopped before the respiration.[11] With a brilliant guess he explained, in part, his own success. "To absence of fear he attributes the favourable statistics of chloroform in childbirth and in operations on young children, and in army hospitals."

Even Edward Lawrie, the most persistent and pugnacious enthusiast of them all, who raised Syme's principles to the rank of an infallible dogma, and who was responsible later for the Hyderabad Commissions' attempts to prove them, and who was, let it be admitted, perhaps the most consistently successful user of chloroform that the world has ever known, had to admit a death.

Discounting his early reference to "thirty or forty thousand cases" because he had obviously not the slightest idea how many anæsthetics he had given up to that time, he did begin to keep exact records of his work in India. This was after he found that people were reluctant to admit the validity of his work on pariah dogs and to accept its value as applied to human beings. Perhaps they were wise enough to think about the effect of cantharides upon the hedgehog! From 1892 to 1899 he reported 14,174 cases, and then he had a death.[12] So the vast population of India gave him an experience much greater than that of his idol, Syme.

It is fairly obvious, then, that anybody, giving chloroform by any method, might easily reach or surpass Syme's total without a death and without any special virtue in the method used.

In the absence of exact information there is always a tendency to over-estimate. If I had been asked to guess the number of anæsthetics I had given over a period of 25 years I should have guessed thirty or thirty-five thousand, quite forgetting the fact that hundreds of long-drawn out operating sessions only increased the number of cases very slowly—quite disproportionately slowly compared to the time they consumed. Having kept a record I know that the correct figure is about sixteen thousand.

That there was a spate of new work is not merely conjecture. It can be proved from the number of hospital operations, which rose to such an extent that it became necessary to have two operating sessions a week instead of one. As early as 1851 *The Lancet* says,[13] while admitting the blessings of anæsthesia:

"It has its drawbacks and evils, amongst the more conspicuous of which may be mentioned the facility with which patients are now persuaded to submit to the knife, and the encouragement which it holds out to what are called 'promising young men' to 'carve their way into practice'. The reports of discussions in the medical societies during the past session are frightfully illustrative of this operating mania."

Syme appears to have had a bee in his bonnet about London and its anæsthesia, judging from his many slighting references to it. At first sight this seems quite irrational. But there was probably a good reason for it—or at any rate a valid reason. In 1848 he was the leading surgeon in Scotland, with more than a national reputation, when, on the death of Liston, he was invited to migrate to University College Hospital. He went to London in February, but in May he resigned his post and returned to Scotland, ostensibly because he was expected to give systematic lectures in surgery in addition to clinical lectures. This reason is commonly given for his resignation, but it does not appear to be a very good one. Surgeons at that time were not—could not be—as busy as they are today. They had no operating lists lasting for hours. They had no elaborate and time-consuming investigations such as cystoscopy or bronchoscopy to do. A few extra lectures could fit easily into their leisured life.

Professor Christison said[14] that Syme's practice in London was a great success, but that he left after two of his colleagues had been grossly insulted by the students without any attempt being made by the governing body to defend them. Was Syme the sort of man, with his world-wide reputation, to need protection? A person with his temper and irascibility was just the man to overawe refractory students. We can be certain that he had no trouble of this sort himself. And he was not the man to resign because his colleagues had had trouble—Syme couldn't care less about his colleagues, judging by his continuous rows with them. It is much more probable that he found that a large fish in a very large pool was not nearly so important as a large fish in a much smaller one—to be exact about one-fourteenth the size.

Slapdash carelessness appears to be the main features of Syme's—or rather Simpson's—method of anæsthesia. No attempt was made to estimate the fitness of the patient; the chloroform was poured on in any quantity by anybody who happened to be available, and very little attempt was made to see what effect it had on the patient. Some of his principles, certainly, are sound—the giving of plenty of air, the watch on the respiration, and the loosening of clothes about the neck. So was the horizontal position and the maintenance of the airway, even though the latter was done by an unnecessarily brutal method. But Syme had no monopoly of these things, as he appeared to think.

In one way, and in one way only, perhaps Syme's teaching was superior to Snow's—in always giving chloroform with the patient lying down. Snow did not attach as much importance to this as he might have done, and gave it in the sitting position in many hundreds of cases. Apart from this, Syme's knowledge of anæsthesia was pitifully inadequate. Snow's grasp of the subject, both theoretical and practical, was far superior, as one would expect. For he was the first whole-time, professional anæsthetist, who gave anæsthetics for an astonishing number of surgeons—he names fifty-two of them, in addition to sixteen dentists and fifteen obstetricians. In considering this astounding feat, which would be quite impossible today, it must be remembered that such things as operating lists lasting for hours simply did not exist. The average operation was completed in five minutes or less, induction time included, and there was no need to waste time on nonsense like washing your hands.

Syme continues his lecture:

In inquiring into the reason of this difference between the experience of chloroform in London and here, we have not far to search for the explanation; it must lie in one of three things—viz., difference in the chloroform, difference in the patients, or difference in the mode of administration; with respect to the chloroform, I believe that most of that which is used in London is made in Edinburgh, and I know that some of the fatal cases might be shown to have occurred with Edinburgh chloroform.

With respect to the patients, it appears that great care is taken in London to use chloroform only in persons free from chest affections, especially cardiac derangements; here we never ask any questions as to the state of the heart or constitution of the patients. In all cases where chloroform is required for an operation. it is freely given. Now, considering the frequency of cardiac disease, and particularly of fatty heart—which, in fact, is I believe rarely absent, at any rate in elderly persons—and considering also, the immense number of patients operated upon, you cannot doubt that many hundreds with fatty degeneration of the heart have had chloroform administered to them here; we even give chloroform without scruple, where we know disease of the heart exists. Within the last week, a case in point occurred in my practice. A patient, with a great dread of pain, and also with a horror of chloroform, had long endured severe pain from his disease, till existence became a burden, because he could not venture to undergo the necessary operation without chloroform, while his medical adviser considered that to take it would be for him almost certain death, on account of organic disease known to exist in the heart; for which he had consulted, and which it may be remarked had been recognised by Dr. Addison, of Guy's Hospital. At length his medical attendant said to him, that he had suffered so much from his complaint, that even if he died under chloroform this would be better than remaining as he was; while, if it should so happen that he should recover, he would be able to enjoy the rest of his life free from the disease. The patient could not resist the force of this argument, and came to Edinburgh prepared for either alternative. I performed the operation under chloroform; and the first thing he did on waking was to ask for a cigar.

As another example, I may mention the case of an old gentleman, aged seventy-four, affected with disease of the heart, from whose bladder I removed a large stone, some years ago. Chloroform was administered as he lay in bed; and he was put so fully under its influence, that he was taken from the bed, was operated upon, and put back to bed, before he woke from his sleep. He recovered perfectly; but some time afterwards died, and Dr. Begbie, on examining the body, found the disease of the heart, which had been diagnosed during life. We cannot, therefore, attribute the absence of deaths here to our being more discriminating than others in the patients to whom we administer chloroform; the very reverse, in fact, being the case.

I think, then, gentlemen, that we are necessarily led to the conclusion, that the difference of results depends on difference in the mode of administration. We know that in other cases differences in the method of procedure have led to differences in results—e.g., it was said in London, that amputation at the ankle invariably causes sloughing; but it turned out that the surgeon who made this statement, performed the operation in a manner that deviated much from the principles on which it is here performed successfully, and which led inevitably to sloughing. So of dividing stricture by external incision, it was said that extravasation of urine must necessarily take place in a dangerous manner, and that other serious complications may occur; but it turned out that the incision had been made without guide on a silver catheter—in short, with such deviation from principles as fully to account for the results.

So far as I can ascertain, from what I have heard and read upon the subject, there are important differences between the mode of administration of chloroform here and in London. It appears that here it is given according to principle, there according to rule.

It is not easy to understand Syme's distinction between principle and

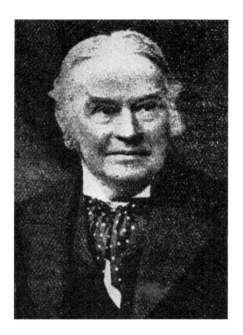

PLATE XXXVI

Brit. med. J., 1908, Jan. 4. 60. Thomas Annandale, Regius Professor of Clinical Surgery, Edinburgh. Born Nov. 2, 1838. Died suddenly Dec. 20, 1907. He succeeded Lister as professor, on the latter's transfer to London.

When a young resident he preserved for us a few valuable statistics of the extent of Syme's operative work. In 1889 (*Brit. med. J., Mar. 2. 465*) he described an oral laryngeal intubation tube as an aid to certain operation. In principle it resembles Kuhn's tube of sixteen years later. In 1897 (*Lancet, Nov. 6. 1184*) he described a tracheotomy tube with an anæsthetic extension.

PLATE XXXVII

Brit. med. J., 1909, June 5. 1360. Lord Lister. Born at Upton, Essex, Apr. 5, 1827. Qualified at University College Hospital in 1852. Worked with Syme for 6 years. Married Syme's daughter, Agnes, 1856. Professor of Surgery, Glasgow, 1869. Professor of Clinical Surgery, Edinburgh, 1869. 1877-1893 Professor of Clinical Surgery at King's College, London. Emeritus Professor until death. Baronet, 1883; Baron, 1897. President of the Royal Society, 1895-1900. Died Feb. 10, 1912. His last surviving house-surgeon, Dr. John Macfee, died in Dec., 1936, aged 92. On Aug. 12, 1865, 71 years before his death, he treated the first compound fracture with carbolic acid by Lister's instructions.

Lancet, 1879, Aug. 16. 246. Sir William Savory criticised Lister's method. He said the best results were obtained by simpler means. "Is it rash to affirm that the future practice of surgery will be most successful when it is carried on, not where antiseptics are most largely used, but under conditions least in need of antiseptics?" Was Savory merely the inevitable obstructionist who always appears as if by magic to oppose new ideas, or had he a faint glimmering of the aseptic methods of the future? I make no attempt to answer this question. This is not a history of surgery.

Lancet, 1938, Nov. 19. 1199. G. Grey Turner. Lister's carbolic spray, which was discarded by 1891, has recently been again brought into use. A young neurological surgeon borrowed one from Turner and used it during prolonged operations to prevent air-borne infection.

The original of this picture had the signature "Lister" under it. It must have been a composite picture. Lister would not use this form of signature until 1897, when he was given the title of Baron. But at that date he was 70 years old, whereas the photograph was obviously taken at least 25 to 30 years earlier.

Lister wrote three articles on Anæsthesia in Holmes and Hulke's *System of Surgery*—mostly in the style of Syme and Simpson, eulogising chloroform and its safety. In the third article, written in 1882, he had to admit a death from it in his own practice.

Lister was a great surgeon—the greatest of all surgeons—and a great man, but why he should be chosen to write on anæsthesia instead of, say, Clover, is beyond all rational comprehension.

Lister succeeded Syme as Professor at Edinburgh, and Sir William Fergusson at King's College—both difficult men to follow, but, of course, his work far outstripped theirs. They were perhaps better technicians than he was, but any advances they could make were merely matters of minor tactics, frequently ruined by their dirty methods, whereas Lister's work altered the whole strategy of surgery and opened up possibilities beyond their wildest dreams. In 1867, when he was at Glasgow, he reported that in nine months not a single case of pyæmia erysipelas or hospital gangrene occurred in his wards, in spite of the fact that they were notoriously unhealthy, being built over hundreds of dead bodies, the victims of a cholera epidemic. He received honorary degrees from 15 universities. He was the first medical peer. Burial in Westminster Abbey was proposed, but he had expressed a wish for Hampstead churchyard.

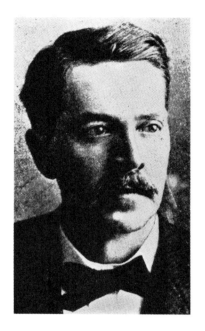

PLATE XXXVIII

Hunter Holmes McGuire. Born 1835. Died at Richmond, Va., Sept. 19, 1900. Chief surgeon of Stonewall Jackson's Army. A great and successful user of chloroform. He had a death from chloroform in 1882. The heart stopped first. This was after about 13,000 cases.

Lancet, 1890, Sept. 27. 684. "To absence of fear he attributes the favourable statistics of chloroform in childbirth and in operations on young children, and in army hospitals." A brilliant and inspired guess.

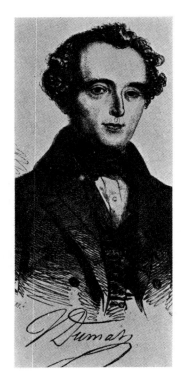

PLATE XXXIX

Lancet, 1851. I. 248. Jean Baptiste Dumas. Born 1800. Chemist. Investigated the chemistry of ether and chloroform. The first to allot a chemical formula to chloroform, incorrect by modern ideas, $C_2 H Cl_3$. Was present at the first operation at the Royal Infirmary, Edinburgh, under chloroform.

rules. Lawrie was also constantly harping on this point, which he regarded as being enormously important. Rightly or wrongly, it appears to me to have very little meaning. For if ever there was a method which could be fairly described as the crudest rule of thumb, it was Syme's. It was something unimportant that students were expected to learn from a ten minute lecture, or from a cursory demonstration on a single case.

There great attention is paid to the number of drachms or minims used; here we are entirely regardless of the amount employed, and are guided only by the symptoms of the patient. The points that we consider of the greatest importance in the administration of chloroform are—first, a free admixture of air with the vapour of the chloroform, to ensure which, a soft, porous material, such as a folded towel or handkerchief, is employed, presenting a pretty large surface, instead of a small piece of lint, or any other apparatus held to the nose. Secondly, if this is attended to, the more rapidly the chloroform is given the better, till the effect is produced; and hence, we do not stint the quantity of chloroform. Then—and this is a most important point—we are guided as to the effect, not by the circulation, but entirely by the respiration; you never see anybody here with his finger on the pulse while chloroform is given. So soon as the breathing becomes stertorous we cease the administration; from what I have learned, it is sometimes pushed further elsewhere, but we consider this in the highest degree dangerous. Attention to the tongue is another point which we find of great consequence. When respiration becomes difficult, or ceases, we open the mouth, seize the tip of the tongue with artery forceps, and pull it well forward; and there can be little doubt that death would have occurred in some cases if it had not been for the use of this expedient. We also always give the chloroform in the horizontal position, and take care that there is no article of clothing constricting the neck. There are thus considerable differences between our practice and that which prevails more or less elsewhere. We use no apparatus whatever, take the respiration as our guide, attend to the condition of the tongue, and never continue beyond the point when the patient is fully under the influence of the anæsthetic.

You observe that in this matter I am very far from taking any credit to myself; all that I have done has been to follow the example of Dr. Simpson, and all that I would say respecting our brethren in London is, that they have not been so fortunate as to get into the right way in the first instance; and I would urge upon them to banish all previous notions, and to keep in view the essential points to which I have alluded; then, if unfortunately there should still be fatal cases, I shall not presume to speak further upon the subject. As the matter at present stands, the discussions prevalent in the profession tend to give the public a dread of chloroform, and to limit the advantages which it possesses, and so long as the differences of opinion seemed due to important differences of practice, I felt called upon to address to you the observations I have made.

"All that I have done has been to follow the example of Dr. Simpson." Syme was not usually so modest. He was a jealous, prejudiced and bad-tempered person, and a superb, though dirty, surgical technician. Of course, all surgeons were dirty at that time.

In 1850 he took legal action against John Lizars, another famous Scottish surgeon, for throwing discredit upon a method of treatment advised by him. He obtained a verdict with costs and damages. In 1866 there was a very acrimonious correspondence in the *Medical Times and Gazette* between Syme and Simpson. The latter thought his use of acupressure to be a very important advance in surgery. Syme did not, and said so publicly in a very rude manner. He quarrelled violently with Liston, and the two were not on speaking terms for years. Not until Liston moved to London, a safe four hundred miles away, did reconciliation take place. His known pugnacity and quarrelsome disposition actually led to his election to the hospital staff being postponed.

A letter reputed to be written by Syme to Liston is worth quoting:[15]

"Dear Liston,—Do you, like some others, believe that I bought the chair of clinical surgery?"

Reply from Liston: "Dear Syme,—If you didn't buy it, how did you get it?"

The same story is given, in a slightly different form in another source. "Dear Syme,—It so happens that I do not know the editor; and if I did, I would not interfere with your lucubrations. How was it, if not by purchase, that you obtained the Chair of Clinical Surgery? Faithfully (signed) Robert Liston. Nov. 8, 1845."[16]

I prefer the first version, for its delightful economy of words, a thing which was very rare in the nineteenth century.

Syme's own account was:

"The truth is that in 1832, Mr. Russell being upwards of eighty . . . requested permission . . . to resign with a retiring allowance from his successor. This request having been granted, Mr. Russell retired, and I became one of three candidates for the vacant chair. In 1833 the late Lord Jeffrey (the Lord Advocate) recommended me for appointment, and I was appointed accordingly."

His patronising attitude to London methods and his superb and arrogant conviction that everything he did was right were not calculated to make him popular.

The supreme assurance with which he made his dogmatic assertions arose from several causes. As he kept no records he no doubt honestly believed that his experience was far larger than it really was. In his complete contempt for figures he fell into the obvious error, as John Snow quickly pointed out, of comparing a small town with a very large one—one nearly fourteen times as big. He possessed the ability to ignore unpleasant or awkward facts which did not fit in with his preconceived ideas—the death which occurred in another part of the hospital, for example. Lastly, owing to the absence of coroners and inquests in Scotland, deaths occurring there were much less likely to be reported in the press, and so arose the legend that nobody ever died of chloroform north of the Tweed.

Syme's ability as a wishful thinker also showed itself in other ways besides anæsthesia. G. Buckstone Browne,[17] in 1901, mentioned that Syme's book on strictures was first published in 1849 and that he died in 1870, thirty-one years before Browne's lecture. "There cannot therefore be many of his patients living now. I have been much interested in meeting professionally with two of them; both died as old men, and both were under my care for tight urethral stricture, showing that the vaunted permanent good results of Syme's external urethrotomy were not always justified by experience." Syme also claimed that he had never known severe hæmorrhage from this operation. Buckstone Browne said that he attended some years ago "a gentleman who some forty years previously had undergone Syme's operation by Syme's own hands . . . he had to pay his Edinburgh landlady three pounds for the mattress, which was ruined by the free bleeding."

There is plenty of evidence from other sources that Syme's attitude was by no means unique. G. H. B. Macleod, surgeon to the Western Infirmary, Glasgow,[18] also gave a clinical lecture on the administration of chloroform in early 1876. He said:

"Free and unrestricted use of chloroform has gone on since 1848; and yet, during those 27 years, no patient has ever died in the operating theatre of either this hospital or the Royal Infirmary from its use. True, four deaths have occurred from chloroform during that time in the latter institution, but they all took place when it was administered for comparatively trivial things in the ward."

Like Syme's case, if death did not occur in the theatre it didn't count, and didn't matter. This lunatic reasoning is all very reminiscent of W. S. Gilbert in reverse. You will remember the dilemma of Ko-Ko, the Lord High Executioner, who described the execution of Nanki-Poo to the Mikado in great detail. A little later he had to explain to the same august and terrifying personage how it came about that the executed Nanki-Poo was still alive.

"When Your Majesty says, 'Let a thing be done,' it's as good as done—practically it *is* done—because Your Majesty's will is law. Your Majesty says 'Kill a gentleman,' and a gentleman is told off to be killed. Consequently that gentleman is as good as dead—practically he is dead—and if dead, why not say so?"

Paraphrased and reversed, the arguments of Syme and Macleod appear to run on similar lines.

I say that no one can die from chloroform, therefore it cannot happen, therefore chloroform is perfectly safe. True, a few misguided individuals, not knowing its perfect safety, have ignorantly died from it, but they ought to have known better. Anyway they only died from trivial operations, not serious ones. When I say a person cannot die he is practically alive, even if he is dead, because he ought not to be dead. And if practically alive, why not say so?

In any case, were these very occasional, reluctantly admitted and 'unimportant' deaths the whole story? In other words, were deaths as rare as these surgeons said? It sounds improbable on the face of it, and in fact it is more than doubtful. There was a medico-legal case years later (in 1903) which throws a vivid light on these guess-work statistics, and on the evil consequences of Syme's doctrines thirty-three years after his death. Professor J. Glaister and Professor H. Galt, both of Glasgow, gave evidence in a case in which damages were claimed for a death under chloroform.[19] The former stated that he had done 30 post-mortems in the last five years on chloroform deaths. The latter had done 13. "We have thus admitted 43 necropsies upon persons dying under chloroform within one district of Scotland."

John Snow's reply to Syme's *ex cathedra* lecture is modest and unassuming. It reveals in a quiet way some of Snow's constant experimental work on the subject, and the depth of his knowledge. There is no evidence that Simpson or Syme ever did any research work at all, except for a few casual and cursory trials of chloroform by Simpson and his assistants during the six days prior to his first public announcement of the discovery. For it was in fact published to the world in less than a week after its very first trial.

Snow did not yet recognise that the early induction deaths were due to chloroform—he considered that they were due to fear alone. But he differentiated clearly between respiratory deaths due to overdosage with a moderate percentage and cardiac deaths due to gross overdose with a concentrated vapour.

He then goes on to point out, quite rightly, that Syme had not considered at all the difference in size between London and Edinburgh, but he does not give any figures himself. This is an omission which ought to be made good. The populations at that time were 3,222,717[20] and 234,550[21] respectively, which means that London could have 13·74 deaths for every death in Edinburgh, and still have the same death-rate.*

Snow is perhaps a little optimistic in saying that overdosage (with a moderately strong vapour) is not possible in the hands of medical men. He overlooked the fact that other doctors had neither his theoretical knowledge, nor his extensive practical experience. They both could and did kill patients with chloroform in every possible way.

Syme was of course quite right in pointing out that no amount of attention to the pulse could give adequate warning of the appallingly sudden cardiac stoppages which caused instantaneous death. Nor could the respiration, for that matter, which Syme considered to be the only true guide. This was a point which he entirely failed to appreciate, as he had been fortunate enough not to come across one of these tragic cases. But he did give the impression that the mere feeling of the pulse was a very dangerous procedure. Lawrie stressed this point even more strongly—to the pitch of absurdity. He implied that feeling the pulse was almost certain to be fatal.

Snow recommends fifteen minim doses of chloroform for analgesia in midwifery. This was the dose he used for Queen Victoria. For anæsthesia he makes the very sensible suggestion of diluting the chloroform with spirit, which at least reduces the chance of overdose considerably. In contrast to Syme's "plenty of air", a somewhat casual and vague statement, Snow gives the percentages needed for safey, worked out in detail by himself.

Lancet (1855), Jan. 27. 108.[22] Reply to Syme's Lecture on Chloroform, by John Snow.

Sir,—I shall be much obliged if you will allow me to make a few brief remarks on the able lecture of Mr. Syme on the subject of chloroform in *The Lancet* of today. I have the happiness to agree with Mr. Syme in the most important points on which he has treated, and if that were all, I should not deem it necessary to address you, for I feel sure that the opinions of this able surgeon would have their due weight, without being endorsed with anything I have to say. It is because I differ from Mr. Syme in some particulars, and because I consider that, in speaking of London as a whole, he has uninten-

*Now, according to *Whitaker's Almanac* (1951 Census), London is 17·87 times as big—for the information of anyone who wants to work out their death-rates.

tionally done an injustice to certain persons, and certain institutions, that I take the liberty of addressing you.

In the first place, however, I wish to state, that I am very much gratified with the remarks of Mr. Syme respecting disease of the heart. There has been for some time such a strong current of opinion, both in the profession and amongst the public, against the administration of chloroform where there is disease of the heart, that I have been almost deterred from repeating my convictions on the subject so strongly as I could wish, for fear of being thought rash and eccentric, and of having my small sphere of usefulness thereby curtailed. If we leave out of view two patients who died suddenly whilst beginning to inhale, and before they could have been affected by the chloroform, and one or two others where the death was most likely unconnected with this agent, I believe that the patients who have died whilst inhaling chloroform have possessed, on the whole, as sound a state of the heart and other vital organs as those who have inhaled it without accident. Persons who require surgical operations are often far from being of sound constitution; and this has been especially the case in my own practice, as patients are often sent to me by medical men who hesitate, or decline altogether to sanction the use of chloroform on their own responsibility. I have found, by very careful observation, that the pain of an operation disturbs the circulation much more, and puts a feeble heart to a much more severe test than chloroform when carefully administered. I have given chloroform, with the most satisfactory result, to very many patients offering all the symptoms of fatty degeneration of the heart in a very marked degree, as the arcus senilis of the cornea, a feeble, intermitting pulse and liability to faint. The only patient I have had the misfortune to lose whilst inhaling chloroform, was, indeed an old gentleman who exhibited the above symptoms in a marked degree. He died as I was proceeding to give a little fresh chloroform, on account of signs of returning sensibility; and I am far from being satisfied that this agent was the cause of his death. The heart was afterwards found to be more degenerated than in many cases where the patient dies suddenly from a very slight shock or exertion, or even without apparent cause.

If the induction of anæsthesia could only be adopted on the strong and robust, it would be a very lame discovery; for persons of feeble or damaged constitution, young children, and the aged and infirm are they who most require to be saved from pain; and again, if the practice could only be advised for extremely painful operations, the patient would be necessarily impressed with an idea of its essential danger, and the greatest benefit connected with the discovery, that of preventing the anxiety and mental anguish arising from the anticipation of an operation, would be altogether lost.

One might perhaps say, paradoxically, that the only justification of the unjustified carelessness of Syme's method was its psychological effect. Supreme confidence in the safety of the drug, whether correct or otherwise, would tend to produce confidence in the patient, which, by lessening his fear—or anxiety and mental anguish, as Snow calls it—would lessen the danger of primary heart failure.

In speaking of London as a place where deaths from chloroform have occurred, and Edinburgh as a place where they have not, Mr. Syme seems entirely to overlook the relative size and population of the two places. When these circumstances are taken into account, the mortality from this cause seems to be pretty equal. At the time the death in Edinburgh occurred, it rendered the mortality of that place higher than in London, and if another death were unfortunately now to occur in Edinburgh, that place would again have the undesirable pre-eminence.

Snow makes the above statements with a sort of quiet confidence, as though he could prove them. But he makes no attempt to do so. How I wished there was some possible means of proving them—or of disproving them, for that matter. My only object was to get at the truth. But how could this possibly be done well over a century later?

Then I remembered that in the course of collecting data and constructing a card index of *anything* in anæsthesia which might by any remote possibility be of historical use, I had photographed, to save writing, a long and detailed table of early chloroform deaths in Snow's book, *Chloroform and other Anæsthetics,* published in 1858. It happened that the photos of this table were too big to be filed in their proper place in the card index, so they had been put away in a drawer and temporarily forgotten.

I got them out, and, to my delight, there were all the facts, set out clearly and unmistakeably. The table, though it no doubt included all the deaths Snow was able to collect, was evidently not complete. Thirty-one of the fifty deaths recorded took place in Great Britain (25 in England and 6 in Scotland), leaving only 19 for the rest of the world. This was obviously so out of proportion as to prove that it was not a complete world list.

Equally obviously, the list was much more likely to be complete as regards Great Britain, the literature of which was easily accessible to John Snow. It is unlikely that any London or Edinburgh case escaped mention, so the figures can be taken as a fairly reliable guide as to the accuracy of Syme's claims for the safety of Edinburgh and the hecatombs of London.

The figures proved Snow's quiet arguments up to the hilt, and gave no support to Syme at all.

Snow's first statement was—"That the London and Edinburgh

mortality is pretty equal." Up to the date of the lecture the score was 13 deaths for London and one for the Scottish capital. So it was on this basis that Syme founded his claim that London "had not got into the right way in the first instance," and kindly offered to put them right. But, it must be remembered, that London at that time was 13·74 times as big as Edinburgh, according to the nearest (1861) Census figures. So it would be difficult to get a more exact equality in the death rate, except by killing fractions of a person.

Secondly, Snow said: "At the time of the Edinburgh death it made the Edinburgh mortality higher than that of London." It did. It practically doubled it at one stroke. Most of the dates are given in the table, and at this time there had been only 7 deaths in London.

His final statement was a prophecy. "If another death were to occur the Edinburgh death rate would be higher again." It did, and it was. When the second Edinburgh death took place the count was London 15 and Edinburgh 2, which meant that the London death *rate* was about half that of the other. The table ceases about two and a half years after Syme's lecture.

It appears then that Syme's basic assumption was wholly without foundation. Perhaps I have been rather hard on Syme in this chapter. But didn't he deserve it?

Snow continues his letter:

If we are reminded that patients go to Edinburgh from a distance, it must be recollected that private patients come here from the East and West Indies, Canada and Australia, expressly for operation, and that hospital patients come from nearly all parts of England and Wales. Chloroform is also administered here in certain cases where the Edinburgh surgeons refrain from its use, as in lithotomy and the removal of tumours of the jaw.

If Mr. Syme alludes only to his own department of the Infirmary, he should not contrast that with the whole of London, for there is at least one hospital here, where a great number of operations are performed, and where no such approach to an accident has occurred as those which Mr. Syme speaks of as having happened in his own practice. In King's College Hospital the breathing of the patient never becomes difficult, or ceases, and it has never been necessary to pull out the tongue with the artery forceps. I have seen faintness in a few patients in this institution from loss of blood during the removal of large tumours with extensive vascular connexions; but I have never had reason to be alarmed on account of the effects of chloroform. The dangers Mr. Syme has incurred have no doubt arisen from his maxim, that "the more rapidly the chloroform is given the better," and I feel certain that under this practice the artery forceps will not always avail to prevent accident. In St. George's Hospital a patient died suddenly whilst beginning to inhale, without being brought under the influence of chloroform, but I believe that there has been no approach to an accident in that institution from the real effects of chloroform. Mr. Syme attributes the supposed greater mortality from chloroform in London to a difference in the mode of its administration, but the real equality in the mortality in the two metropolitan towns is, I think, well explained by the general resemblances of the methods of exhibiting it in both places. In nearly all the cases where accidents have happened in London, the Edinburgh method of exhibiting the chloroform was followed pretty closely. If a piece of lint has been used instead of a handkerchief, or the worsted glove of a dresser, mentioned in Professor Miller's pamphlet, it was, no doubt, because such a slight deviation was not thought of importance.

It is quite true that in certain quarters too great a reliance has been placed on the state of the pulse in administering chloroform, but that is by no means universally the case in London. Indeed, I have only seen a single case in which the person administering the chloroform seemed to rely for his information chiefly on the pulse. I have never heard of an instance where the chloroform was continued when the breathing was stertorous, although of course such an event might occur in a place as large as London without my knowledge. Usually the inhalation is discontinued here as soon as the common sensibility is abolished, without the breathing being rendered stertorous at all. Mr. Syme says that chloroform is given in Edinburgh according to principle, and in London according to rule. It is my opinion that the rules of some of us here proceed from the principles we have taken great pains to ascertain and establish.

Besides the safety of chloroform when carefully administered, and its applicability in all cases of operations, whether there is chest disease or not, there is one other point on which I agree entirely with Mr. Syme—viz., that the vapour of chloroform should be largely diluted with air. I am a little particular and precise on this point, and say that there should never be less than ninety-five parts of air to five parts of vapour. There are two circumstances which I have ascertained to my perfect satisfaction, by very numerous experiments on animals, and what I have observed and heard of the effects of chloroform on the human subject. The first is, that if air containing not more than five per cent. of vapour of chloroform is breathed till the respiration ceases, the heart continues to beat forcibly for some time afterwards. The second is, that when air containing eight to ten per cent. is breathed, it causes a sudden arrest of the action of the heart, by its direct effect on that organ.* Now, although death might undoubtedly take place from a person disregarding the symptoms shown by the patient, and continuing the chloroform too long, such an event has not happened, and is not likely to happen, in the hands of

*There is an asterisk here in the original, but there is no footnote or other reference to it.

161

medical men. All the accidents have been caused by the direct action on the heart of chloroform not sufficiently diluted with air. The pulse has either ceased before the respiration, or about the same time. If a person who has not experimented carefully with chloroform on animals, nor seen a fatal case of its administration, were to judge entirely by his own observation, he would probably conclude that danger began with the respiration (because it is in that function that a very slight overdose manifests its effects when the agent is well diluted with air), but he would be in error.

The first principle in giving chloroform is to ensure that it shall be very largely diluted with air; but the means recommended by Mr. Syme for this purpose are, in my opinion, insufficient to effect it with certainty. The plan I adopt in practice, is to use an inhaler expressly contrived for insuring a very large admixture of air; but I have found that many persons allow an apparatus to get out of order, or they are too careless to consider the express purpose for which it was contrived; therefore, if the use of a handkerchief can be rendered safe, it has many advantages. This can be accomplished in midwifery by putting only fifteen minims (equal to sixty-seven drops) on the handkerchief at a time, and waiting till it is used; but in preparing for a surgical operation, where it is desirable to make the patient quite insensible in about four minutes, it is necessary to use a larger quantity of the agent, and to moisten a greater surface. The proper means to adopt is to dilute the chloroform with spirits of wine. Two parts of spirit and one of chloroform—constituting what Dr. Warren of Boston, United States, calls strong chloric ether—answers very well; but I prefer to use equal parts of chloroform and spirit. The object of the alcohol is not to be inhaled, for it nearly all remains in the handkerchief, but to cause the air to take up less vapour than it otherwise would do. Whilst air is capable of taking up fourteen per cent. of vapour from pure chloroform, at 60° F., it can only take up eight per cent. from chloroform diluted with an equal measure of spirit; and in the practice of inhalation, it would rarely take up more than four or five per cent. from such a solution, and accidents would be avoided.

It has often been repeated, that chloroform is irritating to the air passages when mixed with spirit; but this is altogether a mistake. When chloroform was first administered in London in 1847, it was inhaled from its solution, in about seven parts of spirit, under the name of chloric ether. It produces no irritation whatever, and was only left off on account of the uncertainty of its action in such a diluted form, and its expense. Dr. Simpson, as is well known, afterwards introduced its use in the undiluted state, but except where persons are willing to use a proper apparatus, and take pains with it, it is desirable to return again to a solution of chloroform in spirit, which must be much stronger, however, than that first employed. I am, Sir, your obedient servant, John Snow, M.D.

Sackville Street. Jan., 1855.

His last paragraph is a quiet reproof to Syme's assumption that only in Edinburgh could the Edinburgh-discovered chloroform be given safely—so quiet that Syme probably never noticed it. Snow points out that chloroform was not really a Scottish discovery at all, that it was actually given in London, in spirit, as chloric ether, *before* Simpson introduced its use in the undiluted form. This refers to an incident which is so little known that probably many other people read this letter without noticing it.

But it is an incident not without interest. To get the record straight we will start at the beginning with some rather dull, railway-timetable facts. Three men discovered chloroform almost simultaneously in the year 1831—Samuel Guthrie (1782-1848) of the United States; Eugene Soubeiran in France, and Justus von Liebig (1803-1873), in Germany. It was known as Dutch liquid, chloric ether, bichloric ether or chloride of carbon. Also as perchloride of formyle or chloroformyl. Dumas christened it chloroform in 1834 and gave it the formula C_2HCl_3. It happened, quite by chance, that Dumas was present at the first operation under chloroform at the Edinburgh Royal Infirmary, thirteen years later.

J. P. Flourens used chloroform in animals in 1847, before Simpson used it in humans. R. M. Glover, of Newcastle-on-Tyne, who later gave expert evidence at the inquest on Hannah Greener, had previously (1842) given it to animals *per os* and by injection, but not by inhalation.[23] It was David Waldie, a Liverpool chemist, who suggested its use to Simpson.[24]

And now comes the point which Snow made in such an unobtrusive manner, without mentioning any names at all. Michael Cudmore Furnell wrote a short letter to *The Lancet* in 1871,[25] describing how he used chloroform, in the form of chloric ether, in 1847, six months before Simpson used it. He introduced it to St. Bartholomew's Hospital, where it was used by at least two of the surgeons. His account rings true, because of its modesty. He makes no attempt to dethrone Simpson. Although Furnell did not write this letter until after Simpson died, the story was well known at the hospital and, obviously, well known to Snow. Furnell wrote another letter six years later[26]—a very long one, giving full details of his discovery and adding corroboration from witnesses. But this fits more naturally into another chapter, where the full story can be told.

This was his first short letter:

Sir,—As your columns have been opened to the claims of the rival discoverers of ether as an anæsthetic, perhaps you will allow me to bring to your notice another claimant whose voice has not yet been heard.

Chloric ether (which is chloroform plus spirits of wine) was first administered to produce insensibility during a surgical operation at St. Bartholomew's Hospital by Mr. Holmes Coote, to a patient of Sir William (then Mr.) Lawrence, at my recommendation, in the spring of 1847. I was a pupil at the time, and had just commenced my studies at St. Bartholomew's. Trying the effects of sulphuric ether, which as your correspondent, "An American," justly says was introduced by Dr. Morton of Boston, United States, I by accident came to try chloric ether, a preparation then little used. The effect in producing insensibility was found to be exactly the same as sulphuric ether, while it was free from the disagreeable taste which made sulphuric ether so suffocating to most people. At Mr. Jacob Bell's recommendation, I took some with me to St. Bartholomew's, and brought it to the notice of Mr. Holmes Coote, who was then Mr. Lawrence's assistant. On my assuring him that I had tried it on myself, and that it was perfectly safe, it was administered by him to one of the hospital patients, who was about to be operated upon that very day, and its success was so decided that Mr. Lawrence subsequently administered it with complete success to a lady who was unable to take sulphuric ether.

My object in placing these facts on record is in no way to detract from the fame of the great physician (Sir James Simpson) who has just left us. Far from it. To him, I believe, belongs the merit of having recommended, or at any rate, introduced, to the profession the use of chloric ether minus its spirits of wine—i.e., chloroform. But it seems to me and many of my friends worth placing on record, amongst the numerous claimants who have now sprung up, the fact that chloric ether, which is almost chloroform, was first used as an anæsthetic in our oldest London Hospital by one of its most famous surgeons.

Your obedient servant, M. C. Furnell, F.R.C.S., Surgeon, H.M.'s Indian Army. Professor of Physiology, Madras Medical College. February, 1871.

Holmes Coote was therefore prepared for Simpson's revelation, and it is not surprising that he was one of the very early users of chloroform itself in London.[27] On Saturday, Nov. 20th, 1847, only ten days after the first local publication of the news in Edinburgh, and the very day of its first publication in *The Lancet*, he operated on three cases under the new drug, which had been made by Mr. Taylor, of Vere Street. It was given by Mr. Tracy, who had already designed an ether apparatus, on a thin flat sponge. The first case was a lithotomy—the induction took two minutes, the operation seventy-five seconds. Another lithotomy followed, this time induced in less than one minute, but the operation was slightly slower at ninety seconds. The third operation was a tumour of the breast, a long case, which took three minutes. (Now you see why John Snow was able to work for such a fantastic number of different surgeons.)

Coote's comment was "some modification in the mode of its administration may be requisite, since, as I am informed by Mr. Mitchell Henry, one of the house surgeons, the lips of two of the patients have been vesicated by the application of the sponge."

The battle between Syme and Snow led to later repercussions in the following numbers of *The Lancet*. Supporters of both Tweedledum and Tweedledee voiced their opinions. R. R. World[28] complained:

"It is hard of the learned professor to say that all his brethren in this large town 'have not been so fortunate as to get into the right way in the first instance.' Let me assure Mr. Syme that not all his London brethren who administer chloroform require a grim assistant physician, with watch in hand, to take charge of the pulse."

Mr. World's own experience in the last seven years was upwards of 4,000 cases—about twice that of Syme himself—and he had had no anæsthetic deaths. He added that he found the insensibility of the eye to touch and light useful as an indicator of the depth of anæsthesia. He agreed that free mixture with air was essential, and stated that he could regulate this with the apparatus he used, but he does not name this. He ended by saying that he attached much importance to the quality of the chloroform. Mr. Syme did not appear to consider this. Is all chloroform made in Edinburgh good?

Mr. James Arnott, the enthusiastic advocate of refrigeration anæsthesia by means of crushed ice and salt,[29] said that few people would agree with Syme about the unimportance of heart disease in chloroform cases. To kill another patient by chloroform for the extraction of a toenail, for instance (already there had been four deaths from this cause), would now, as the public was fully aware of its danger, be considered culpable homicide. Arnott thought that many chloroform deaths in private practice were not reported.

A letter signed Hopewell, Edinburgh,[30] states emphatically that the pulse is observed during anæsthesia in London, in spite of John Snow's denials. Mr. Erichsen, in his *Science and Art of Surgery*, advises that "During the whole time it is the duty of the administrator to keep his hand on the pulse."

Three months later Mr. Arnott is at it again.[31] Both the rapid Edinburgh method and the slow method, he says, quite correctly, have caused fatalities. He reports that chloroform has been prohibited at the Massachusetts General Hospital. Fatalities may be expected to be greater in private practice owing to lack of hospital facilities for resuscitation, but private practice deaths are less likely to be published.

One or two earlier references have a bearing on the controversy. In 1849[32] Syme admitted that he had opposed Simpson's view that anæsthesia protected patients from shock, but had now changed his mind and was convinced that Dr. Simpson was right in his opinion.

Snow stated in his letter that Edinburgh surgeons did not use chloroform in certain difficult cases, such as jaw and tongue operations, whereas this was not the case in London. In 1851, four years before, Mr. Fergusson[33] removed the right mandible under chloroform given by Snow himself. He kept the anæsthesia going by means of a sponge. "This case might seem decisive as to the propriety of using chloroform in operations upon the face; and it certainly appears that apprehensions are far too anxious in this respect."

This was not an isolated case, for the year after *The Lancet* comments:[34]

"it should not remain unmentioned that chloroform is now extensively given in operations upon the face and mouth. We saw Mr. Erichsen, at University College Hospital, a few days ago, remove a portion of the tongue whilst the patient was under the influence of the anæsthetic agent. By nice management, and keeping a sponge impregnated with chloroform steadily under the nose, the unconscious state may be kept up for a long period."

Snow, in these cases, gave the anæsthetic in a sitting position, kept the patient very lightly under so that the cough reflex was present, and tilted the head forward from time to time to clear the mouth of blood. These precautions could be carried out successfully by a skilled anæsthetist, who knew exactly how deep an anæsthesia he wanted and how to keep it at the required level, but they were obviously impracticable when the chloroform was given by raw students, as was Syme's invariable practice. This led to anæsthesia being withheld in these cases when they were dealt with by Syme's obsolete method, which was antiquated even at that date.

In 1864, no less than seventeen years after the first use of chloroform,[35] Syme performed a particularly brutal and horrible operation. On November 29th he began by extracting a tooth, then cut through the lower lip, sawed through the mandible, tied the lingual arteries and removed the whole tongue in two pieces. It was a case of carcinoma.

The horrible thing about it was that all this protracted torture was done without anæsthesia of any kind; "since the patient, instead of lying horizontally, might thus be seated in a chair, so as to let the blood run out of his mouth. . . ."

Syme was, of course, quite right in assuming that anæsthesia in a case of this sort was quite beyond the capacity of an unskilled student. But surely, in seventeen years, he might have learnt that even cases of this kind could be, and were, tackled successfully by a few experts. Snow had done it thirteen years earlier.[36]

But in the cocksure ignorance of his omniscience Syme held fast to his opinion that chloroform could be given by anybody, and if it couldn't it was just too bad. The idea that any improvement in his crude method could ever be made—had in fact been made—was completely beyond him.

REFERENCES

1 *Lancet* (1855), Jan. 20. 55.

2 *Lancet* (1904), Jan. 9. 77. J. B. Hellier.

3 *Brit. med. J.* (1870), Feb. 26. 199. A case of sudden death in ovariotomy while the patient was under the influence of chloroform. By Sir James Y. Simpson.

4 *Lancet* (1855), Dec. 8. 560.

5 *Lancet* (1855), Dec. 8. 560.

6 *Lancet* (1849), Feb. 24. 205.

7 *Lancet* (1855), Jan. 20. 55.

8 *Lancet* (1862), Dec. 6. 623.

9 *Lancet* (1861), Jan. 26. 98.

10 T. Holmes and J. W. Hulke. *A System of Surgery* (1883). 3rd ed. Vol. III. (pp. 598-624).

11 *Lancet* (1890), Sept. 27. 684.

12 E. Lawrie. *Chloroform.* London. J. and A. Churchill.

13 *Lancet* (1851), Jan. 11. 54.

14 *Lancet* (1870), Dec. 10. 830.

15 *North Briton* (1858), Mar. 20. Original reference not checked, but it makes a good story.

16 *Mon. J. med. Sci.* (Edinb.: 1846). Vol. VI.

17 *Lancet* (1901), Nov. 30. 1476.

18 *Brit. med. J.* (1876), Jan. 1. 4.

19 *Lancet* (1903), April 25. 1183.

20 1861 *Census. Population Tables. England and Wales* (1862). Vol. I, p. 224. Eyre and Spottiswoode.

21 1861 *Census of Scotland. Figures supplied by the National Library of Scotland.* Royal City and Burgh. 66,429. Parliamentary Burgh. 168,121.

22 *Lancet* (1855), Jan. 27. 108.

23 *Edinb. med. surg. J.* (1842). No. 152. Not verified.

24 *Lancet* (1847). II. 687.

25 *Lancet* (1871), Mar. 25. 433. M. C. Furnell, M.D., F.R.C.S., Surgeon-Major, H.M.'s Indian Service.

26 *Lancet* (1877), June 30. 934. M. C. Furnell.

27 *Lancet* (1847), Nov. 27. 571.

28 *Lancet* (1855), Feb. 3. 141.

29 *Lancet* (1855), Feb. 10. 169.

30 *Lancet* (1855), Feb. 17. 187.

31 *Lancet* (1855), May 12. 496.

32 *Lancet* (1849), Mar. 3. 236.

33 *Lancet* (1851), May 17. 545.

34 *Lancet* (1852), Nov. 6. 425.

35 *Lancet* (1865), Feb. 4. 115.

36 *Lancet* (1851), May 17. 545.

INDEX

Roman figures = plate numbers.

Arabic figures = page numbers.

INDEX

INDEX